Dedication

To my wife Sultana, and for our children, Suja and Asmi

Table of Contents

Preface

The subject of anatomy is very vast. An attempt to write a complete book on anatomy is an overwhelming undertaking. By breaking this tremendous project down into smaller steps, it can be completed more efficiently and effectively. "Thoracic Anatomy Tutor" is the first step in reaching that goal.

The volume of material generally taught from any anatomy text books is very large and can be troubling to a new student, particularly to a student with no previous experience to adequately prepare them for the examination. It can be difficult for a novice student to match the level of more experienced peers and disappointment due to poor grades on examinations may be frustrating. A wonderful subject like anatomy may become a nightmare and studying more like drudgery. An anatomy textbook is full of information, but may not have sufficient examples of questions to focus the student's study. It has been found that solving questions immediately after studying a topic is conducive for long-term memory and attaining the highest scoring on examinations. For proper conception, both multiple choices questions and objective questions solving are vital. "Thoracic Anatomy Tutor" is designed to meet these demands.

The approaches to the study of anatomy are changing. Problem Based Learning (PBL) with case studies is emphasized in today's curriculum. Anatomy students today are the doctors and health care professionals of the future and it is expected that they will solve clinical challenges utilizing the anatomical knowledge gained during their education. The duration of a gross anatomy course and method of evaluation are variable from region to region. Gross anatomy is taught for about two years in medical colleges of Indian subcontinents, sixteen weeks in medical schools in the United States, and fourteen weeks in the medical schools of the

Caribbean. Gross anatomy is extensively taught in the chiropractic colleges, but also focused upon in dental, nursing, physical therapy and occupational therapy programs. A student of any of these programs needs an easy to follow, amiable book with all the relevant, up-to-date information required for health care professional of today. The concept is further clarified if the gross anatomy is learned along with the relevant embryology and histology, because they are interlinked.

"Thoracic Anatomy Tutor" is written for the average students at any level of learning.

I am obliged to my wife Dr. Bahar Sultana. Her continuous inspiration guided me all through. My son D.M. Suja helped me in computer set ups for the figures.

I admit that there might be errors within the book in spite of repeated proof reading. Any suggestions to improve the book are encouraged and appreciated. Please put your suggestions through e-mail at dewanraja@hotmail.com

Sincerely,

Dewan S. Raja, MBBS, M Phil, MPH,CPH, CHES.,
DTM&TH

Thorax

Overview

The **thorax** is the part of the trunk between the root of the neck and the diaphragm. The **trunk** consists of the thorax and abdomen, which includes the pelvis. The thorax contains and protects the principal organs of respiration (*lungs*) and circulation (*heart*), and part of the alimentary tract (*esophagus*). It also contains the followings: lower part of the trachea; bronchi; major blood vessels (*aorta, superior and inferior vena cava, azygos vein*); lymphatic vessels like thoracic duct; nerves (*intercostal, thoracic sympathetic trunk, splanchnic nerves*); nerve plexuses (*esophageal, cardiac and pulmonary plexuses*). The thorax communicates with the root of the neck at the superior thoracic aperture (*thoracic inlet*) and is enclosed by the diaphragm at the inferior thoracic aperture (*thoracic outlet*).

Clinician vs. Anatomist and "Thoracic Outlet Syndrome"

Anatomists describe the *superior thoracic aperture* as the *thoracic inlet* because air and food enter the thorax only through this aperture. Clinicians tell describe the superior thoracic aperture as the *thoracic outlet* because the arteries and T1 spinal nerves emerge from the thorax through this aperture to enter the lower neck and upper limbs. In **thoracic outlet syndrome**, the emerging structures are affected by obstruction. Thoracic outlet syndrome is a clinical condition caused by compression of the nerves and or blood vessels between the neck and shoulders. **The lower trunk of the brachial plexus (C8, T1), together with the subclavian vessels** may be compressed or angulated over a cervical rib. The patient may present with **vascular symptoms** (ischemic pain) due to subclavian artery kinking and is associated with a large bony cervical rib. **Neurological deficits** (tingling, numbness, paraesthesia, and weakness) may also be present and associated with small rudimentary cervical rib, which extends into a fibrous band and joins the superior surface of the first rib interiorly. Thoracic outlet syndrome is manifested by slow onset of wasting of small muscles of the hand. The pain of thoracic outlet syndrome is often aggravated by carrying heavy objects.

Superior thoracic aperture

The *superior thoracic aperture* (anatomical thoracic inlet) is bounded anteriorly by the superior border of the manubrium sterni, posteriorly by the first thoracic vertebral body and laterally by the first pair of ribs and their costal cartilages. It is kidney shaped (reniform) and because of the obliquity of the first pair of ribs, the aperture slopes anteroinferiorly. In an adult male the superior thoracic aperture is approximately 6.5 cm anteroposteriorly and 11cm transversely.

Inferior thoracic aperture

The *inferior thoracic aperture* (anatomical thoracic outlet) and is bounded anteriorly by the xiphoid process, anterolaterally by the costal margin (formed by the costal cartilages of ribs (7-12), posteriorly by the body of the 12th thoracic vertebra, and posterolaterally by the 11th and 12th pairs of ribs.

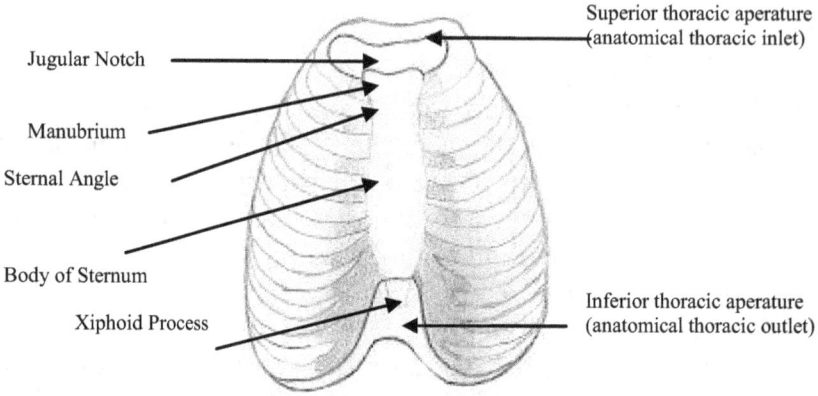

Thoracic apertures

The **dome of the diaphragm** may rise to the level of the fourth intercostal space, and the abdominal viscera, including the liver, spleen and part of the stomach, lie superior to the plane of the inferior thoracic aperture, within the thoracic wall.

The **thorax** is bounded anteriorly by the sternum, posteriorly by the body of the 1st to 12th thoracic vertebrae, and laterally by the 1st to 12th ribs and their costal cartilages.

 Bony cage of the thorax is formed by the sternum, twelve pairs of ribs and costal cartilages, and twelve thoracic vertebrae. The bony cage supports and protects the thoracic viscera. The bones of the **thoracic cage** have a significant cancellous part which produces blood cells (hematopoeisis). The bony cage also assists in respiration.

Axillary folds
The pectoralis major and overlying skin forms the *anterior axillary fold*. It bridges the thoracic wall to the humerus and bounds the axilla anteriorly. The *posterior axillary fold* is formed by the latissimus dorsi, teres major and overlying skin. It bounds the axilla posteriorly.

Table: Position of the thoracic structures according to the vertebral levels

T2/T3	Jugular Notch (Suprasternal Notch)
T3/T4	Arch of the Aorta
T3	Root of the spine of the scapula
T4/T5	Manubriosternal Junction (Angle of Louis or Sternal Angle)
T5	Thoracic Duct Crosses the Midline (From Right to Left Side of the Vertebral column)
T7	Inferior Angle of the Scapula
T8	Vena Cavil Opening of the Diaphragm (Transmits Inferior Vena Cava and

	Branches of the Right Phrenic Nerve)
T9	Xiphisternal Joint
T10	Esophageal Opening of the Diaphragm (Transmits esophagus, Anterior and Posterior Vagal Trunks, and Left Gastric Vessels)
T12	Aortic Opening of the Diaphragm (Transmits Aorta, Thoracic Duct, Occasionally Azygos and Hemiazygos Vein)
L1	Tip of the 9th costal cartilage
L3	Lowest part of the costal margin

Rib levels

Superior angle of the scapula   2nd rib
Inferior Angle of the scapula   7th rib

Important Dermatomes

Clavicle   C3, C4
                           (Supraclavicular nerves)
Xiphoid process   T6
Nipple (male and female)   T4

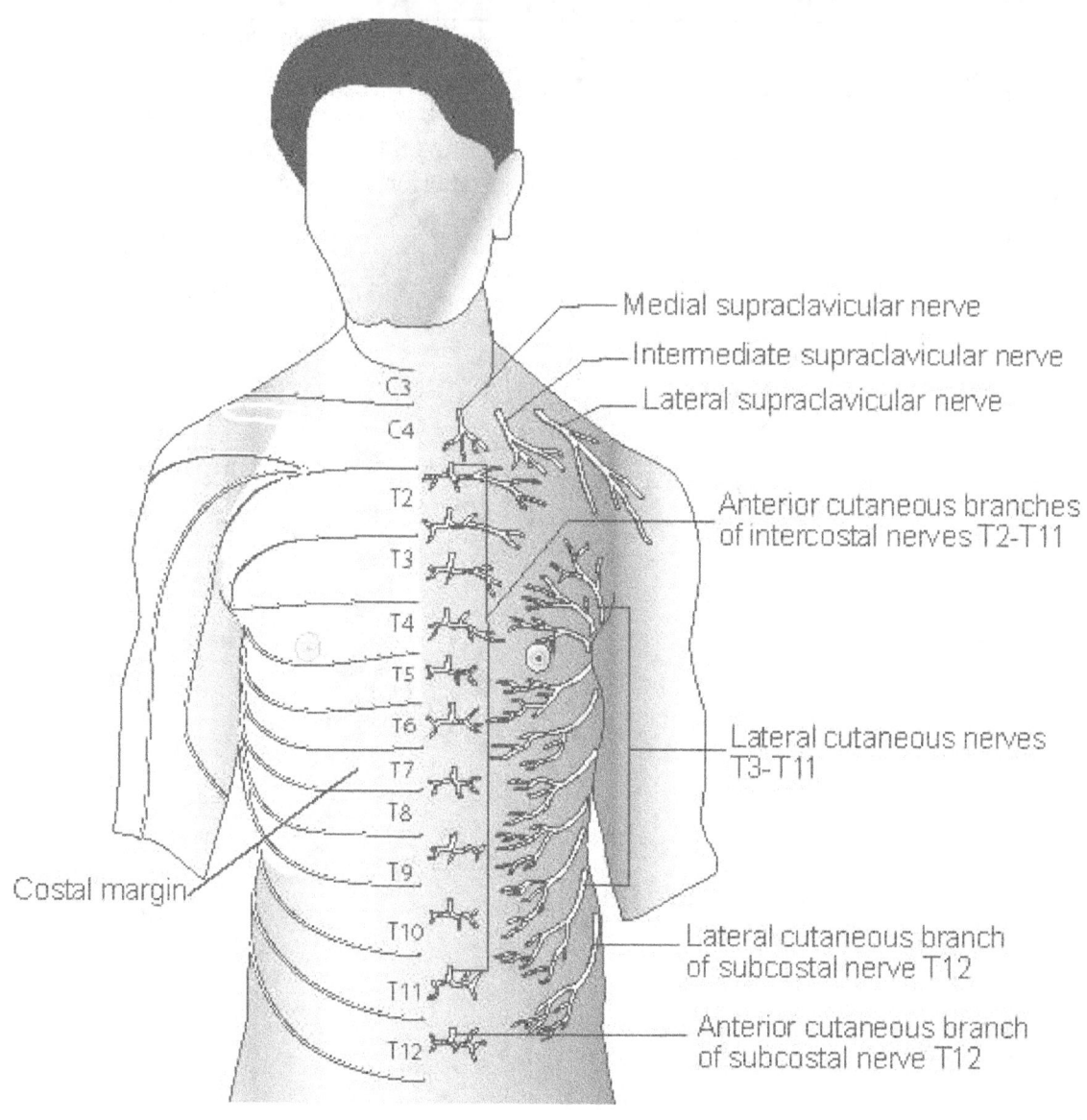

Figure: Dermatomes and cutaneous nerves of the thoracoabdominal region

Objective Questions (Set-1)
1. Define trunk.
2. Define thorax.
3. Define chest.
4. What is Thoracic Outlet Syndrome?
5. What are the boundaries of the thorax?
6. What is the boundary of the superior thoracic aperture?
7. What is the boundary of the inferior thoracic aperture?
8. How are axillary folds formed?
9. Which is larger, the thorax or chest?
10. What Structures are present/cross at the vertebral level of T4/T5, T5, and T2/T3?
11. How is the bony cage of the thorax formed?

Multiple Choice Questions (Set-1)
1. Functions of the bony cage of the thorax include _____.
   A. Attachment of the trachea
   B. Attachment of the lungs
   C. Attachment of the base of the heart
   D. Support and protection of the viscera

2. Which of the following structures passes through the vena caval opening of the diaphragm?
   A. Superior vena cava
   B. Left gastric vessels
   C. Esophagus
   D. Anterior and posterior vagal trunk
   E. Branches of the right phrenic nerve

3. Which of the following muscles contributes in the formation of the posterior axillary fold?
   A. Pectoralis major
   B. Pectoralis minor
   C. Teres major
   D. Teres minor
   E. Deltoid

MCQ (Set-1) Answers: 1. D; 2. E; 3. C

Thoracic cavity and the mediastinum

The thoracic cavity is subdivided into three major compartments, which include two **pleural cavities** (left and right) each surrounding a lung and the **mediastinum**. The mediastinum is a mass of tissue between the two pulmonary cavities. It is a thick, flexible soft tissue partition oriented longitudinally in a median sagittal position inside the thoracic cavity that contains the pericardium, heart, esophagus, trachea, major blood vessels, and nerves. The mediastinum acts as the partition between the lungs and includes the mediastinal pleura, which extends vertically from the thoracic inlet to the diaphragm.

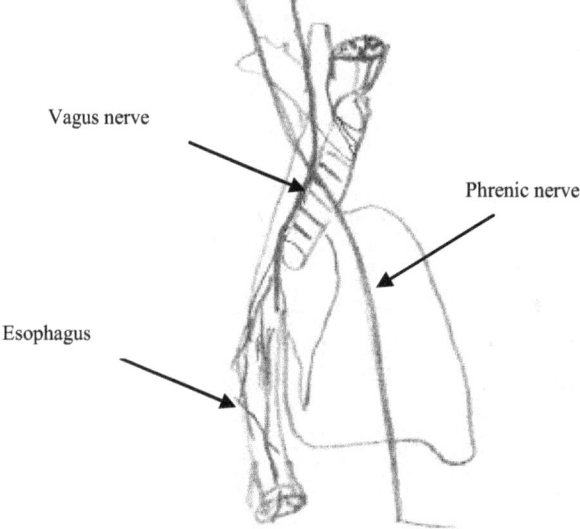

Vagus nerve

Phrenic nerve

Esophagus

Vagus & Phrenic nerve

Classification/location and contents of the mediastinum

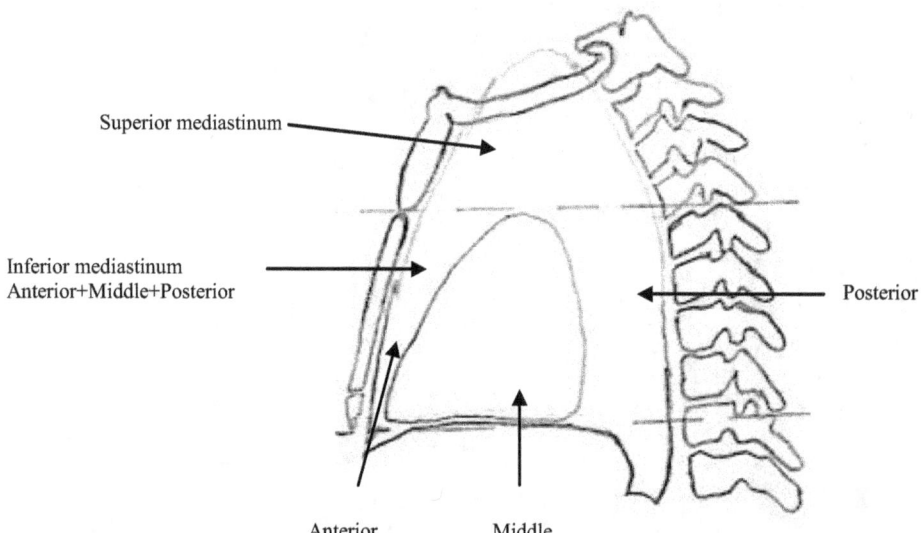

Superior mediastinum

Inferior mediastinum
Anterior+Middle+Posterior

Posterior

Anterior   Middle

Superior mediastinum is the mediastinum (partition between the lungs) that lies above the horizontal plane that extends from the angle of Louis (manubriosternal angle) to the lower border of the 4th thoracic vertebra. This horizontal plane is often referred to as the transverse thoracic plane.

Inferior mediastinum is the mediastinum that lies below the horizontal plane that extends from the angle of Louis to the lower border of the 4th thoracic vertebra (transverse thoracic plane). The inferior mediastinum has three components: *middle mediastinum; anterior mediastinum; and posterior mediastinum.*

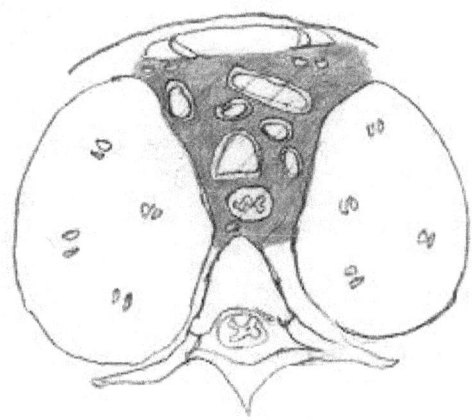

Superior mediastinum (shaded area)

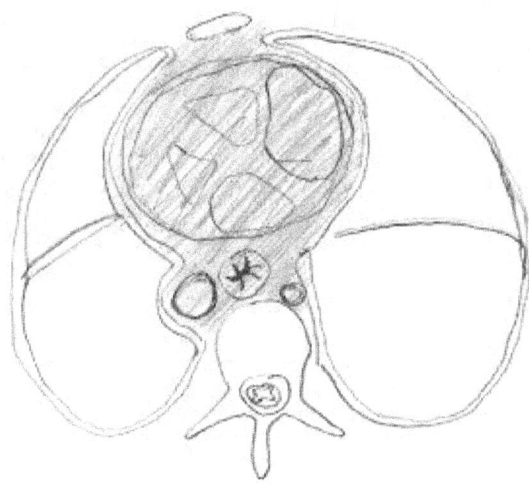

Inferior mediastinum (shaded area)

Superior Mediastinum

Boundaries	Contents
Anteriorly: Manubrium sterni Posteriorly: T1 to T4 thoracic vertebrae Superiorly: Plane of thoracic inlet Inferiorly: Transverse thoracic plane Laterally: Mediastinal pleura	1. Trachea and esophagus 2. Arteries: arch of the aorta and its branches 3. Muscles: origin of sternothyroid; sternohyoid; and longus colli 4. Veins: right and left brachiocephalic veins; upper part of superior vena cava; and left superior intercostal vein 5. Nerves: vagus nerve; phrenic nerve; cardiac nerves; left recurrent laryngeal nerve 6. Thymus 7. Thoracic duct

Middle Mediastinum

Boundaries	Contents
Anteriorly: Anterior mediastinum Posteriorly: Posterior mediastinum Superiorly: Transverse thoracic plane Inferiorly: Central tendon of the diaphragm Laterally: Mediastinal pleura	1. Heart with pericardium 2. Arteries: ascending aorta; pulmonary trunk; and left and right pulmonary arteries 3. Veins: terminal part of the azygos vein; inferior half of superior vena cava; and right and left pulmonary veins 4. Nerves: left and right phrenic nerves; deep cardiac plexus 5. Inferior tracheobronchial lymph nodes 6. Bifurcation of the trachea 7. Left and right primary bronchi

Anterior Mediastinum

Boundaries	Contents
Anteriorly: Posterior surface of the body of the sternum Posteriorly: Pericardium Superiorly: Transverse cervical plane Inferiorly: The diaphragm Laterally: Mediastinal pleura	1. Sternopericardial ligaments 2. Mediastinal branches of the internal thoracic artery 3. Lower part of the thymus (sometimes) 4. Lymph nodes 5. Loose connective tissue

Posterior Mediastinum

Boundaries	Contents
Anteriorly: Middle mediastinum Posteriorly: T4 to T12 vertebrae Superiorly: Transverse cervical plane Inferiorly: The diaphragm	1. Artery: descending thoracic aorta and its branches 2. Veins: azygos; hemiazygos; accessory hemiazygos vein 3. Nerves: vagus and splanchnic nerves 4. Esophagus 5. Thoracic duct 6. Posterior mediastinal lymph nodes

Structures passing through more than one mediastinum

The *esophagus* passes through both the superior and posterior mediastinum. The esophagus begins from the lower end of the laryngopharynx in the neck and ends in the stomach in the abdomen.

The *vagus nerve* passes through the superior and the posterior mediastinu. It begins in the brainstem and ends in the junction between right 2/3 and left 1/3 of the transverse colon.

The *phrenic nerve* passes through the superior and middle mediastinum. The phrenic nerve is formed by vental rami of C3, C4, and C5 spinal nerves and ends on the under surface of the diaphragm and gall bladder.

The *thoracic duct* passes through posterior and superior mediastinum. It is formed in the abdomen and ends at the root of the neck at the junction between the left internal jugular vein and left subclavian vein.

Additional notes
- An infection present in the neck behind the prevertebral fascia (a part of deep cervical fascia) cannot go beyond the superior mediastinum because the prevertebral fascia is attached to the T4 vertebra.
- An infection present between the pretracheal and prevertebral fascia can reach the posterior mediastinum because the pretrachael fascia blends with the arch of the aorta.
- The pleural cavity, also known as the pulmonary cavity, is not included in the mediastinum.
- There are two pleural **cavities** left and right; each cavity contains a lung.
- The diaphragm is a partition between the thorax and the abdomen. The diaphragm is a sheet of skeletal muscle with a triangular central tendon.
- Thorax consists of the thoracic **cavity**, its contents, and the wall that surrounds it.
- Shape and size of the thorax are smaller than those of the chest
- The chest includes the thorax and parts of the upper limb bones and muscles, and mammary glands.
- Pleural cavities are completely separated from each other by the mediastinum.
- Abnormal events in one pleural cavity does not necessarily affect the other cavity.
- The mediastinum can be entered surgically without opening the pleural cavities.
- Pleural cavities extends above the level of the 1st rib.
- The apex of each lung actually extends into root of the neck.
- Abnormal events in the root of neck can involve adjacent pleural and lung and vice versa.

Objective Questions (Set-2)
1. Define mediastinum.
2. Classify mediastinum.
3. Describe the boundaries of the superior mediastinum, the inferior mediastinum, the anterior mediastinum, and the middle mediastinum.
4. What are the contents of middle mediastinum, anterior mediastinum, posterior mediastinum, and superior mediastinum?
5. What structures are present in more than one mediastinum?
6. What is mediastinal syndrome?
7. Why the infection behind the prevertebral fascia cannot reach the posterior mediastinum?
8. Why is the infection behind the pretracheal fascia can reach the posterior mediastinum?
9. What is the transverse thoracic plane?

Multiple Choice Questions (Set-2)
1. The posterior mediastinum contains_____.
   A. Sternopericardial ligaments
   B. Ascending aorta
   C. Heart
   D. Phrenic nerve
   E. Esophagus

2. Which of the following structures may be compressed by a malignant tumor of the posterior mediastinum?
   A. Trachea
   B. Esophagus
   C. Ascending aorta
   D. Left Brachiocephalic vein
   E. Brachiocephalic trunk

3. Which of the following structures is present in the middle mediastinum?
   A. Esophagus
   B. Descending thoracic aorta
   C. Pericardium
   D. Azygos vein
   E. Vagus nerve

4. Which of the following structures is present in the anterior mediastinum?
   A. Azygos vein
   B. Esophagus
   C. Descending thoracic aorta
   D. Vagus nerve
   E. Sternopericardial ligaments

5.   Select an INCORRECT statement about the transverse thoracic plane:
   A. It separates the superior mediastinum from the inferior mediastinum.
   B. Anteriorly it goes through the angle of Louis.
   C. Posteriorly it goes through the Intervertebral disc between the T4-T5.
   D. It separates the anterior mediastinum from the posterior mediastinum.

6.   Which of the following structures is present in both the superior and middle mediastinum?
   A. Vagus nerve
   B. Phrenic nerve
   C. Esophagus
   D. Azygos vein
   E. Descending thoracic aorta

MCQ (Set-2) Answers: 1. E; 2. B; 3. C; 4. E; 5. D; 6. B

Functions of the thorax
1. Breathing - the diaphragm, flexible thoracic wall, the ribs, the lungs and the work together.
2. Protection of the vital organs - protects the heart, lungs and great vessels.
3. Conduit - the mediastinum acts as a conduit for structures that pass through the thorax from the neck to the abdomen.

Structures passing through the inlet of the thorax
- **Viscera**: trachea, esophagus, apices of the lungs and remains of the thymus.
- **Large vessels**: brachiocephalic trunk, left common carotid artery, left subclavian artery, right and left brachiocephalic veins
- **Nerves:** right and left phrenic nerves, right and left vagus nerves, right and left sympathetic trunks, right and left first thoracic nerves
- **Muscles**: Sternohyoid, sternothyroid and longus colli

Cervical rib
A *cervical rib* is the costal element of the **C7**. It may be a mere epiphysis on its transverse process or have a head, neck, tubercle and shaft. It occurs in about 0.5% of subjects and is rarely associated with symptoms. The posterior end of the cervical rib is attached to the C7 vertebra. The anterior end of the cervical rib is attached to the 1st rib, 1st costal cartilage, or rarely to the sternum.

Thymus
The *thymus* is a lymphoid organ and is responsible for thymus processed lymphocytes, which is essential for **cell mediated immunity.** The size of the thymus is at its largest up to the age of 15, then it involutes gradually although persists actively into old age. It is **located** in the root of the neck, superior and anterior mediastinum. *Hassal's corpuscles* are whorls of concentrically layered epithelial cells, present in the medulla of the thymus. The thymus is supplied by the **internal thoracic vessels**.

Development of the thymus
The lymphocytes are derived from mesoderm. The epithelial **reticular cells** are derived from the endoderm, from the **3rd pharyngeal pouch**. Epithelial reticular cells maintain the *blood thymus barrier*. *Hassall's corpuscles* are seen in the medulla of the thymus and their number **increases with the aging process**. Hassall's corpuscles are formed from the accumulation and degeneration of the epithelial reticular cells. Hassall's corpuscles are rich in keratin and sometimes calcified. The function of the Hassall's corpuscle is unknown at this time.

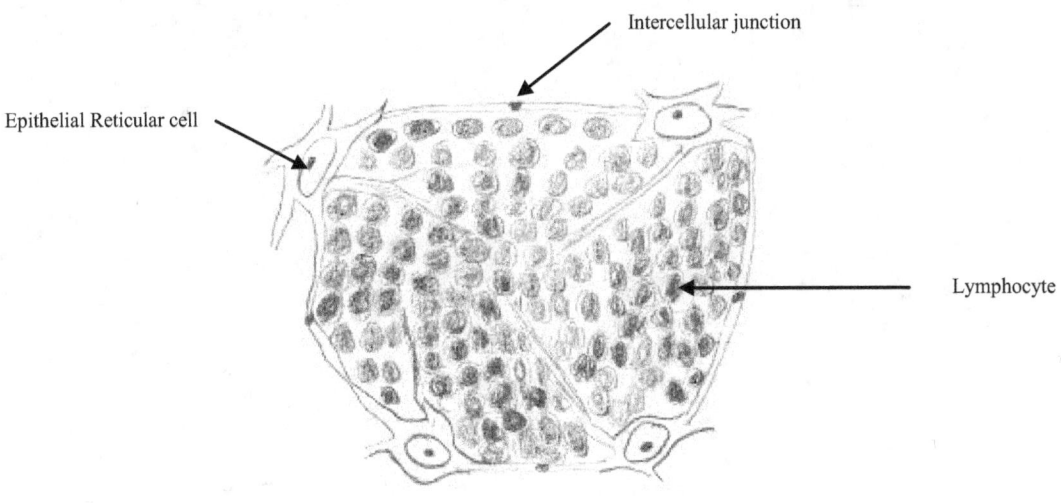

Epithelial Reticular cell

Intercellular junction

Lymphocyte

Histology of Thymus gland

Thymoma

Thymoma is a tumor of the thymus gland and may be associated with myasthenia gravis. Thymoma may be a cause of thoracic outlet syndrome. **Myasthenia gravis** is a disorder of the neuromuscular junction due to acetylcholine receptor abnormality. It is characterized by fatigue and exhaustion. *Thymoma* (a mostly benign tumor) is associated with 30% of the cases of myasthenia gravis. Thymectomy, removal of the thymus, is the treatment in those cases.

DiGeorge's syndrome

The congenital absence of the thymus gland is called DiGeorge's syndrome. Patients with this disease cannot produce T cells. They have lack cell-mediated immunity and hence die at an early age.

Scalene muscles

There are three scalene muscles. They are the *anterior scalene, middle scalene* and *posterior scalene*. Scalene muscles take origins from the transverse process of the cervical vertebra. Scalenus anterior and medius are inserted into the 1st rib. Scalene posterior is inserted into the 2nd rib. Scalenus minimus is an extension of the scalenus anterior and not considered a fourth independent muscle.

Suprapleural membrane (Sibson's fascia)

Suprapleural membrane is an extension of the **endothoracic fascia**. The endothoracic fascia is a thin layer of loose connective tissue that separates the costal pleura from the thoracic wall. Suprapleural membrane reinforces the cervical pleura and resists changes in intrathoracic pressure occurring during respiratory movements. This prevents any distention of the root of the neck during respiration. *Suprapleural membrane* is attached laterally to the medial border of the first rib and first costal cartilage; posteriorly to the apex of the transverse process of the seventh cervical vertebra; and medially to the fascia investing the structures passing through the thoracic inlet. The suprapleural membrane is also called the tendon of the scalenus medius.

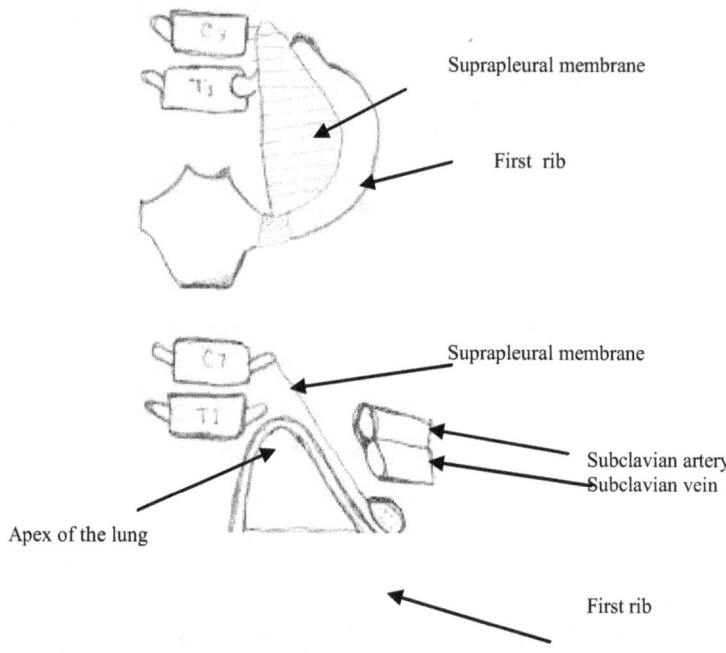

Suprapleural membrane

Objective Questions (Set-3)
1. From which germ layers does the thymus gland develop?
2. What type of cells form the blood-thymus barrier?
3. What is the usual location of a thymus gland in a 12 year old boy?
4. What is thymoma?
5. What is Hassall's corpuscle?
6. How is Hassall's corpuscle formed?
7. What is the function of the thymus?
8. What is Sibson's fascia?
9. What is endothoracic fascia?
10. What are functions of the suprapleural membrane?
11. What are the attachments of the suprapleural membrane?

Multiple Choice Questions (Set-3)
1. A 23-year old soldier received shrapnel wound over the left clavicle in Iraq by the explosion of an IED. Recently, during a physical examination, it was revealed that when he blew his nose or coughed, the skin above the left clavicle bulged upward. The skin was bulging due to a defect in which of the following structures?
   A. Suprapleural membrane
   B. Cervical pleura
   C. Prevertebral fascia
   D. First rib

MCQ (Set-3) Answers: 1. A

Bones of the Thorax

Sternum

The *sternum* is a flat bone which forms the anteromedial part of the **thoracic cage**.

The sternum consists of three parts, the *manubrium, body (mesosternum)* and *xiphoid process (xiphisternum)*. The sternum contains highly vascular *trabecular bone* (spongy bone) which is sandwiched by the compact bone. Trabecular bone contains red bone marrow. The upper part of the sternum is called manubrium. Bone marrow is collected from the manubrium for pathological studies. This collection is called a ***sternal biopsy***. Sternal biopsy is indicated to diagnose blood dyscracia, metastatic cancer, and to identify some parasites. The ***jugular notch*** is present on the superior margin of the sternum bounded bilaterally by the lower end of the sternocleidomastoid muscle. The sternum is innervated by the supraclavicular nerve, intercostal nerve, and phrenic nerve.

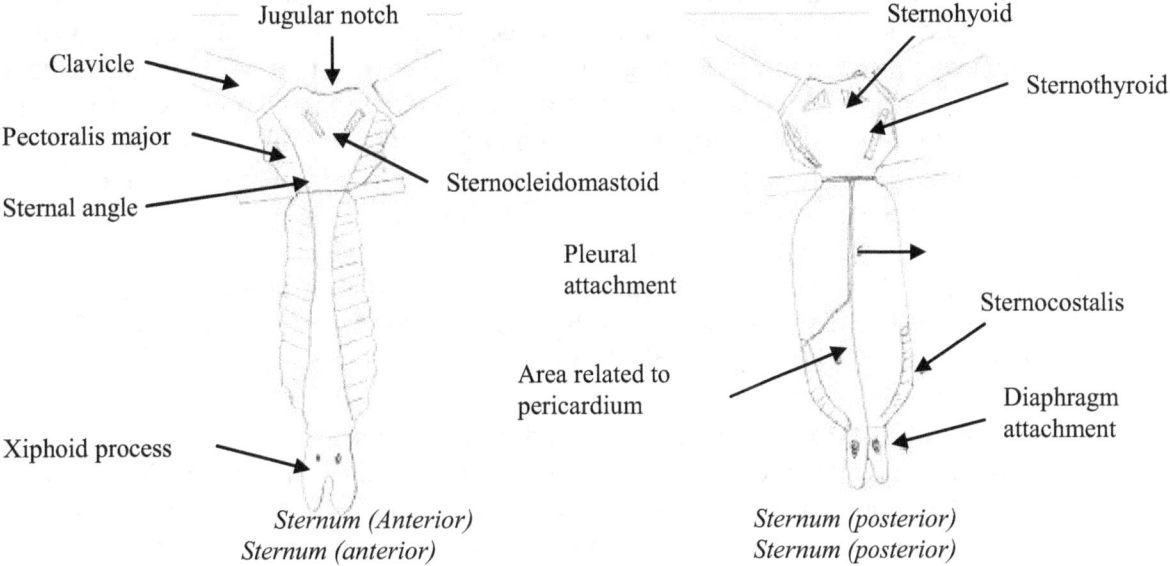

Sternum (Anterior)
Sternum (anterior)

Sternum (posterior)
Sternum (posterior)

Sternal angle

The *sternal angle* is also called the *manubriosternal angle* or the ***angle of Louis***. This is the angle between the manubrium and the sternal body (mesosternum). Sternal angle is indicated by the bony ridge and palpated easily. Costal cartilages and ribs can be counted from the sternal angle. The 2nd costal cartilage articulates with sternum at the angle of Louis.

Relations to the sternal angle level:

1. Intervertebral disc between the T4 and T5 vertebrae
2. The 2nd costal cartilage articulates with the sternum at the sternal angle. So, the ribs can be counted easily.

3. Aortic arch begins and ends
4. The trachea bifurcates into right and left principal bronchus
5. The azygos vein opens into the superior vena cava
6. The superior vena cava penetrate the pericardium to enter the heart.
7. Superior limit of the pulmonary trunk

The **body of the sternum** is at the level of the **T5-T9** vertebra. The mesosternum articulates with the 2nd to 7th costal cartilages. The mesosternum articulates with the xiphoid process at xiphisternal joint. Xiphisternal joint is at the level of the T9 vertebra. The intermammary furrow in an adult female overlies the skin over the mesosternum. Sometimes a sternal foramen is found in the lower part of the sternum due to lack of ossification and does not bear any significance.

Xiphoid process
The *Xiphoid process* is at the level of **T10** vertebra. It is the lowest tapering part of the sternum. In infancy it is cartilaginous but in adult it is ossified. The Xiphoid process is variable and can be broad and thin, pointed, bifid, perforated, curved or deflected. The 7th costal cartilage articulates to the xiphoid process. It can be palpated in the upper epigastrium. The linea alba is attached to the lower end of the xiphoid process. The **dermatome** over the xiphoid process is T6. The xiphoid process lies in a slight depression in the epigastric fossa, where the converging costal margins form the infrasternal angle. This angle is used in cardiopulmonary resuscitation **(CPR)** for locating the proper hand position.

The following structures are present at the level of the xiphisternal joint: infrasternal angle; superior limit of the liver in the midline; central tendon of the diaphragm; inferior border of the heart.

Muscles attaching to the posterior surface of sternum
Two muscles attach to the posterior surface of the manubrium sterni. They are the *sternohyoid* and the *sternothyroid*. The *transverse thoracis (sternocostalis)* is attached to the posterior surface of the body of the lower sternum. Attachment to the posterior xiphoid surface is made by muscular slips of the diaphragm.

Muscles attaching to the anterior surface of the sternum
Two muscles attach to the anterior surface of the manubrium sterni. They are the *pectoralis major* and *sternocleidomastoid* muscles. The *pectoralis major* is also attached to the anterior surface of the body of the sternum. The attachment to the anterior surface of the xiphoid process is by the medial fibers of the rectus abdominis, the aponeurosis of external oblique, and the aponeurosis of internal oblique. The border of the xiphoid process also gives attachments to the aponeurosis of internal oblique, aponeurosis of transversus abdominis, and the upper end of the linea alba.

Ectopia cordis
In ectopia cordis, the heart protrudes outside the chest through a split in the sternum. In other forms the heart may be situated in the abdominal cavity or neck. Associated defects are the rule and death often occurs at the first day of life.

Treatment, in those whom it is possible, is surgical and involves covering the heart with skin and repairing or palliation of associated defects.

Notes:

1. Sternotomy is carried out for open heart surgery.

2. The sternum may be fractured due to its subcutaneous location

3. Bone barrow is aspirated from manubrium sterni to diagnose certain diseases(e.g.,leukemia).

4. A horizontal plane passing through the sternal angle separates the superior mediastinum from the inferior mediastinum

Content of the deltopectoral triangle (bounded by deltoid, pectoralis major and clavicle)

The deltopectoral triangle contains terminal part of the **cephalic vein**. The cephalic vein opens into the axillary vein.

Thoracic vertebrae

Each thoracic vertebra has two *costal facets on each side of the body*, also known as *demi facets*. The body of each thoracic vertebrae is typically heart shaped. The facets are present on the transverse processes for articulation with the tubercle of their respective ribs. The normal convexity of the thoracic segment of the vertebral column is directed posteriorly.

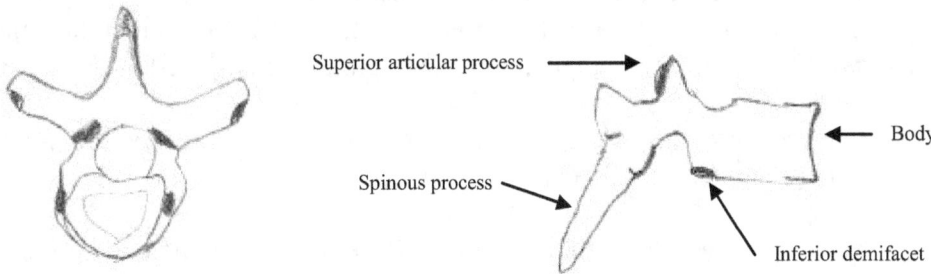

Typical thoracic vertebra superior view view   *Typical thoracic vertebra lateral*

The thoracic vertebral canal contains the *spinal cord* and *meninges*. The contents of the thoracic vertebral canal can be exposed by a surgical procedure called a *laminectomy*. A section of lamina is removed revealing a window into the canal.

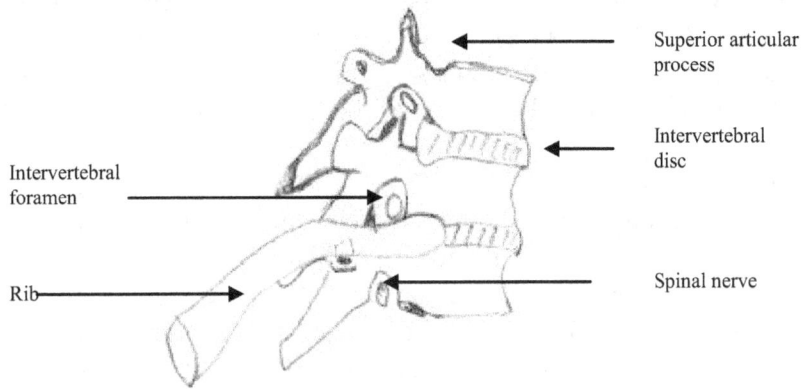

Section of thoracic vertebral column, intervertebral disc, intervertebral foramen with spinal nerve and rib

Ligaments of the thoracic vertebrae
1. Anterior Longitudinal Ligament
2. Posterior Longitudinal Ligament
3. Ligamentum Flavum
4. Supraspinous Ligament
5. Interspinous Ligament
6. Intertransverse Ligament

Differences between the thoracic vertebrae from the lumbar and cervical vertebrae
The thoracic vertebrae have costal facets. The cervical vertebrae have transverse foramina. The lumbar vertebrae have neither costal facets nor transverse foramina. The lumbar vertebrae have mammillary and accessory processes.

Muscular attachment of the thoracic vertebra
There are three muscles attaching to the thoracic vertebral body. They are the *longus colli*, which arises from the T1, T2, and T3 vertebral bodies, the *psoas major*, and the *psoas minor*, both originating from the 12th thoracic vertebra.

Intertransverse, levatores costarum, and deep dorsal muscles are attached to the transverse process of the thoracic vertebra.

Seven muscles attach to the spinous process of the thoracic vertebra. They included the *trapezius, rhomboid major* and *minor, latissimus dorsi, serratus posterior superior, serratus posterior inferior* and deep dorsal muscles are attached to the spinous process of the thoracic vertebra. The *rotator* muscle attaches to the posterior aspect of the lamina of the thoracic vertebra.

Convexity of the thoracic vertebrae
Normal convexity of the thoracic segment of the vertebral column is directed posteriorly
Excessive curvature of the thorax in the sagittal plane (forward bending) is called *kyphosis*. **Kyphosis** is seen in older patients and may be due to degeneration of vertebral body and intervertebral discs, secondary deposits of cancer in the vertebral column, or tuberculosis of the thoracic vertebral body (Pott's disease).

Ribs
The ribs are long, slender elastic arches which form a large part of the skeleton of the thorax. Ribs structurally consist of highly vascular trabecular (spongy) bone enclosed in a thin layer of compact bone. The trabecular part of the bone contains red bone marrow. Ribs are flat bones and are a component of the axial skeleton. There are typically twelve pairs of ribs (with eleven intercostal spaces), but the number may be increased by cervical or lumbar ribs or reduced to eleven by the absence of the last pair of ribs. The **longest** of all the ribs are the 7th pair. All the

ribs are attached posteriorly to the thoracic vertebrae at the costovertebral joints. The 8th, 9th, and 10th ribs do not reach the sternum and they form most of the costal margin (vertebrochondral ribs). The two costal margins are easily palpable and they extend inferolaterally from the xiphisternal joint. The costal margins form the sides of the infrasternal angle. The costal margins are fomed by the 7th, 8th, 9th and 10th ribs.

The chest wall of a child is very elastic and fractures of ribs in children are rare.

Types of ribs
There are different types of ribs, which include typical ribs, atypical ribs, floating ribs, and true ribs. The 11th and 12th ribs are called *floating ribs* or *vertebral ribs* because the anterior ends are unattached and free floating. The first two and last three pairs of ribs present special features and are called *atypical ribs*. *True ribs* (*vertebrosternal ribs*) are the upper seven pairs of ribs because the costal cartilages articulate with the sternum. *False ribs* are the 8th to 12th ribs because they are not directly connected to the sternum.

Parts of a typical rib
The costal end articulates with the costal cartilage. The vertebral end articulates with the costal facets of the thoracic vertebrae. The tubercle of the rib has an articular surface that forms a joint with the transverse process of the corresponding vertebra. The shaft is the long portion of the bone. **The angle of the rib** is the apex of the curve in the rib. The vertebral end of a typical rib articulates in three areas; the superior costal facet of the corresponding vertebra; the inferior costal facet of the one vertebra above; and the intervertebral disc between the corresponding vertebra and one vertebra above.

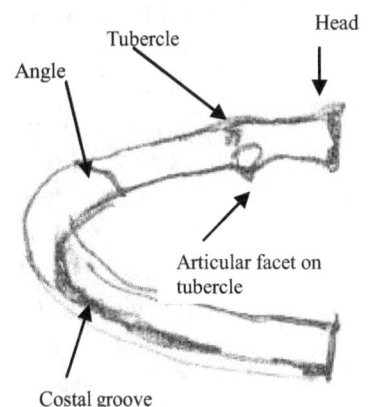

Typical left rib, posterior view

Costal groove
The costal groove is on the internal surface of the shaft of the rib. It is located just above the lower border, running along the length of the shaft. Within the groove, from above downward, are the intercostal vein, the intercostal artery, and the intercostal nerve. The **mnemonic** is "V A N."

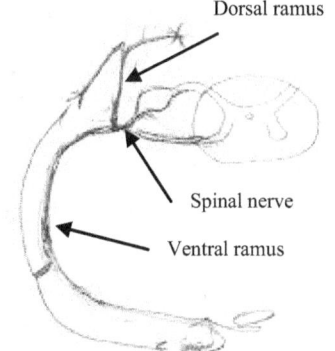

Typical intercostal nerve

First rib
The first pair of ribs is the shortest, stoutest, and most curved of all the ribs. There is no costal groove. The head of the first rib articulates with the first thoracic vertebral body only. The superior surface of this rib is marked by two

shallow grooves separated by the scalene tubercle to which scalenus anterior is attached. Anterior to the scalene tubercle is the groove for the subclavian vein. Posterior to the scalene tubercle is the groove for the subclavian artery. The first rib is not palpable because it is deeply located and is covered by muscles.

Flail chest

When multiple ribs are fractured, each in two or more places, a movable segment of the thoracic wall **(flail chest)** is produced. There will be paradoxical movement of the thoracic wall occurs during respiration. During inspiration, the flail segment moves in and during expiration

the flail segment moves out .Flail chest may affect ventilation and may require assisted ventilation.

Joints of the thorax

There are different types of joints within the thorax. The sternoclavicular joint provides the only bony attachment between the appendicular and axial skeletons. It has a fibrocartilaginous articular surface and contains two separate synovial cavities.

Sternoclavicular	saddle type synovial joint
First sternocostal	primary cartilaginous joint
2nd to 7th sternocostal	synovial plane joints
Costochondral	primary cartilaginous joints
Costovertebral	plane type of synovial joints
Costotransverse	plane type of synovial joints
intervertebral discs	symphysis, secondary cartilaginous joint
Interchondral	plane type of synovial joint
Manubriosternal	secondary cartilaginous joint
Xiphisternal	primary cartilaginous joint

Blood supply of the thoracic vertebrae
Arterial supply

Posterior intercostal artery, branch of descending thoracic aorta provides blood supply to the thoracic vertebrae. On each side, the main trunk of the posterior intercostal artery passes around the vertebral body, giving of periosteal and equatorial branches to the body, and then a large dorsal branch. The dorsal branch gives off a spinal branch which enters the intervertebral foramen, before itself supplying the zygapophyseal joints, the posterior surface of the laminae and the overlying muscles and skin. The spinal branch divides into three branches, prelaminar, radicular, and postcentral branches and enters inside the vertebral canal through the intervertebral foramen. The postcentral branches are the main nutrient arteries to the vertebral bodies and the intervertebral disc, epidural tissue and duramater. The prelaminar branch supplies the vertebral arch, the posterior epidural tissue, duramater and the ligamentum flavum. The radiculer branch supplies the spinal cord and nerve roots. There are rich anastomoses among the branches of the arteries.

Venous drainage

Veins of the thoracic vertebrae include external and internal venous plexuses and basivertebral vein. The basivertebral vein drains venous blood from the vertebral body, comes out through the posterior foramina of the vertebral bodies. All groups are devoid of valves, anastomose freely with one another, and join the intervertebral veins. The intervertebral veins emerge through the intervertebral foramen accompanying the spinal nerves. The intervertebral vein drains to the brachiocephalic veins above and azygos system of veins below.

Objective Questions (Set-4)

1. What structures are related to the posterior surface of the manubrium sterni?
2. What structures are present at the level of the xiphisternal joint?
3. What muscles are attached to the xiphoid process?
4. What structures are related, begin, and end at the level of the sternal angle?
5. What are the parts of a typical thoracic vertebra?
6. What ligaments are attached to a typical thoracic vertebra?
7. What muscles are attached to a typical thoracic vertebra?
8. How can you differentiate a thoracic vertebra from a cervical and a lumbar vertebra?
9. Why is a laminectomy done?
10. What is Kyphosis? What is Scoliosis?
11. What is Lordosis?
12. Which ribs are false ribs?
13. Which ribs are true ribs?
14. Which ribs are floating ribs?
15. Which ribs are atypical ribs?
16. Which ribs are typical ribs?
17. With how many vertebrae does a typical rib articulate?
18. Which rib has scalene tubercle?
19. Which structures pass in front of and behind the scalene tubercle?
20. Which ribs are related to the spleen?

Multiple Choice Questions (Set-4)

1. Which of the following bones is located in the median plane of the anterior wall of thorax?
   A. Clavicle
   B. Scapula
   C. 1st rib
   D. Sternum

2. Which of the following muscles has attachment to the body of the sternum?
   A. Sternohyoid
   B. Sternohyoid
   C. Transversus thoracis

D. Sternocleidomastoid

3. The 2nd costal cartilage can be located by palpating the
   A. Jugular notch
   B. Costal margin
   C. Angle of Louis (sternal angle)
   D. Xiphisternal angle
   E. 1st costochondral joint

4. Which of the following events/landmarks does not occur at the sternal angle?
   A. Trachea bifurcates into left and right principal bronchi.
   B. Coronary arteries originate from the ascending aorta.
   C. Azygos vein opens into the superior vena cava.
   D. Border between superior and inferior mediastinum.
   E. Superior border of the fibrous pericardium

5. The jugular notch is bounded laterally by the:
   A. Pectoralis major
   B. Pectoralis minor
   C. Longus colli
   D. Sternocleidomastoid

6. Which of the following costal cartilages is connected to the xiphoid process?
   A. 5th costal cartilage
   B. 6th costal cartilage
   C. 7th costal cartilage
   D. 8th costal cartilage
   E. 9th costal cartilage

7. Which of the following is the dermatome over the nipple of a lactating mother?
   A. T2
   B. T3
   C. T4
   D. T5
   E. T6

8. The arch of the aorta is related to which of the following?
   A. Manubrium sterni
   B. Mesosternum
   C. Sternoclavicular joints
   D. Middle third of the clavicle

9. Which of the following costal cartilages does not articulate with the body of the sternum?

A. 1st costal cartilage

B. 2nd costal cartilage

C. 6th costal cartilage

D. 7th costal cartilage

10. Which of the following costal cartilages forms the costal margin?
   A. 1st and 2nd costal cartilages
   B. 3rd and 4th costal cartilages
   C. 5th and 6th costal cartilages
   D. 7th, 8th, 9th and 10th costal cartilages
   E. 11th and 12th costal cartilages

11. Which of the following abdominal organs is lacerated due to fracture of the left 10th rib?
   A. Fundus of the stomach
   B. Left kidney
   C. Left suprarenal gland
   D. Spleen
   E. Left lobe of the liver

MCQ (Set-4) Answers: 1. D; 2. C; 3. C; 4. B; 5. D; 6. C; 7. C; 8. A; 9. A; 10. D; 11. D

23

Pleura

The pleura is a double layer, thin, serous membrane that consists of *parietal pleura* and *visceral pleura*. The pleura facilitates smooth movement of the lungs. The visceral pleura covers the lungs and the parietal pleura lines the inner surface of the thoracic wall. The potential space between the visceral and parietal pleura is called the **interpleural space, pleural cavity, or pleural sac**. There is always slight negative pressure in the interpleural space, which keeps the lungs inflated. Both the parietal and visceral pleura are lined by simple squamous epithelium. The visceral pleura is closely adhered to the lungs and can not be dissected from the lung. The parietal and visceral pleura are continuous at the hilum of the lungs.

Simple Squamous Epithelium

The *parietal pleura* is divided into four parts. The *thoracic pleura* lines the ribs. The *cervical pleura,* also called *pleural cupula*, extends through the superior thoracic aperture into the neck and extends 2.5 cm above the medial end of the clavicle at the root of the neck. The *diaphragmatic pleura* covers the superior surface of the diaphragm. The *mediastinal pleura* covers the lateral aspects of the mediastinum and includes the *pulmonary ligament*.

The *parietal pleura* is supplied by the nerve, artery, and vein of the body wall (somatic) because it develops embryologically from the somatopleuric mesoderm. The *visceral pleura* is supplied by the nerve, artery and vein of the lungs because it develops from the splanchnopleuric mesoderm. Normally the pleura secretes a few milliliters of serous fluid, which allows for ease of movement for the lungs during inspiration and expiration.

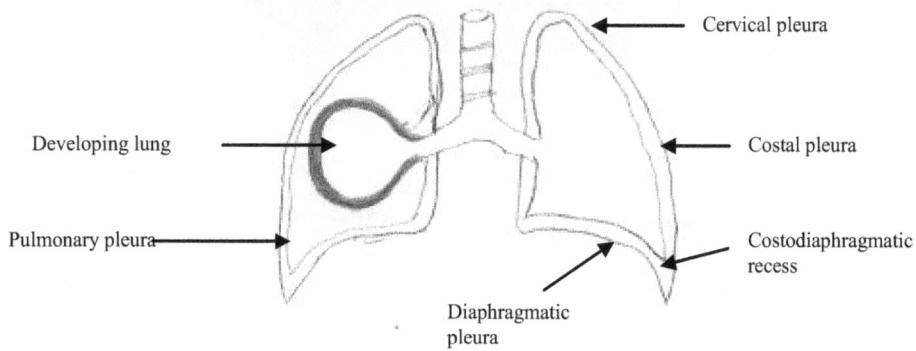

Lungs and pleural

In pleural effusion, the interpleural cavity may contain in excess of 1-3 liters of fluid. This is commonly due to pulmonary tuberculosis or chronic heart failure. Presence of pus or purulent fluid in the pleural space is called *empyema thoracis*. Air in the pleural space is called *pneumothorax* and may be due to stab injury or rupture of congenital cyst. The presence of both fluid and air in the pleural cavity is called *hydropneumothorax*.

The fluid in the pleural cavity settles in the *costodiaphragmatic recesseses* in an ambulatory patient

Percussion of the thorax
In a healthy individual, percussion on the chest wall gives a tympanic sound. In pleural effusion, percussion on the chest wall gives stony dull sound.

Pleurisy and pleural rub
If the visceral pleura lacks the lubrication to smoothly move with the parietal pleura, a rubbing noise is heard upon auscultation called pleural rub. The *pleural rub* will be heard rhythmically with breathing. *Pleurisy* is a dry form of inflammation without a significant collection of fluid in the pleural cavity.

Recesses of pleura
There are two folds or recesses of parietal pleura which act as reserve spaces for lungs to expand during deep inspiration. The *costomediastinal recesses* lie anteriorly, behind the sternum and costal cartilages, between the costal and mediastinal pleura. The *costodiaphragmatic recesses* are the space between the diaphragmatic pleura and the costal pleura. Vertically the costodiaphragmatic recesses measures about 5cm, and extends from 8th to 10th ribs along the midaxillary line. **Fluid accumulates first** in the costodiaphragmatic recesses in pleural effusion. In **emphysema**, which is a chronic lung disease in which the bronchioles are permanently dilated, the costodiaphragmaic recesses are very distinct.

Pulmonary ligament
The mediastinal pleura surrounding the root of the lung extends downward beyond the root as a fold called the *pulmonary ligament*. The fold contains a thin layer of loose areolar tissue with a few lymphatics. The pulmonary ligament provides a dead space into which the pulmonary veins can expand during increased venous return, such as during exercise. The lung roots can also descend into the pulmonary ligament as the diaphragm descends.

Innervation of the pleura
The costal and peripheral parts of the *diaphragmatic pleura* are innervated by the *intercostal nerves*. The mediastinal pleura and central part of the diaphragmatic pleura are innervated by the *phrenic nerve*. The *pulmonary pleura* is innervated by the same autonomic nerves as the lung, which include the sympathetic from the T2 to T5 spinal segments and parasympathetic innervation through the vagus nerve. Parietal pleura is pain sensitive while the visceral pleura is not.

Blood supply and lymphatic drainage of the parietal pleura
The parietal pleura is supplied by the *intercostal*, *internal thoracic* and *musculophrenic arteries*. The venous blood from the parietal pleura drains into the *azygos* and *internal thoracic veins*. The lymphatics from the parietal pleura drain into the intercostal, *internal mammary*, *posterior mediastinal* and *diaphragmatic lymph nodes*.

Blood supply and lymphatic drainage of the visceral pleura
The *visceral (pulmonary) pleura* gets arterial blood from the *bronchial arteries*. The venous blood from the *pulmonary pleura* is drained into the *bronchial veins*. Lymph from the visceral (pulmonary) pleura is drained into the *bronchopulmonary lymph nodes*.

Reflection of the pleura on the thoracic wall
These are the lines along which the *parietal pleura* passes (reflects) from one wall of the pleural cavity to another. The *sternal line of pleural reflection* occurs when the costal pleura becomes continuous with the mediastinal pleura anteriorly. *The costal line of pleural reflection* is also sharp and occurs where the costal pleura becomes continuous with the diaphragmatic pleura inferiorly. *The vertebral line of pleural reflection* occurs where the costal pleura becomes continuous with the mediastinal pleura posteriorly.

The pulmonary pleura along the inferior border of the lung is two ribs above the parietal pleura along the costodiaphragm recesses.

Extension of the parietal and visceral pleura
Anteriorly
- the pleura extends from the sternoclavicular joint to reach the midline at the sternal angle, the pleura deviate to the left at 4th costal cartilage (cardiac notch) arches back at 6th costal cartilage
- the pleura deviates to the right at 6th costal cartilage
- the visceral pleura reaches rib 6 at the mid-clavicular line
- the parietal pleura reaches rib 8 at the mid-clavicular line

Laterally
- the visceral pleura (inferior border of the lung) reaches rib 8 at the mid-axillary line
- the parietal pleura reaches rib 10 at the mid-axillary line

Posteriorly
- the visceral pleura (along the inferior border of the lung) reaches rib 10
- the parietal pleura reaches rib 12

Thoracocentesis
Thoracocentesis is the process of removal of pleural fluid from the pleural cavity by inserting a hypodermic needle through an intercostal space. Thoracocentesis is carried out through **9th intercostal space in the midaxillary line during expiration** to avoid injury to the inferior border of the lungs. Thoracocentesis is done to remove fluid, blood or pus from the pleural cavity. **A needle will encounter the following structures in order**: skin; superficial fascia; external intercostal muscle; internal intercostal muscle; innermost intercostal muscles; parietal pleura.To avoid damage to the intercostal nerve and vessels, the needle is inserted superior to the rib, high enough to avoid the collateral branches. When the patient is in upright position, interpleural fluid is accumulated in the costodiaphragmatic recess.

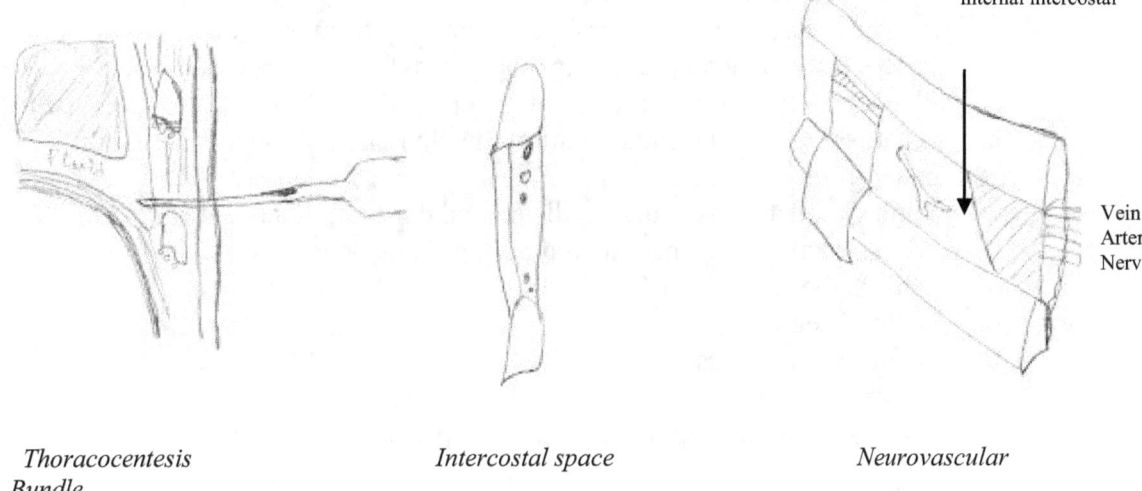

Internal intercostal

Vein
Artery
Nerve

Thoracocentesis Bundle   *Intercostal space*   *Neurovascular*

Pectus excavatum

Pectus excavatum (*funnel chest*) is a depression of the sternum and costal cartilages that results in a funnel shaped chest. Pectus excavatum is usually linked with **lordosis and or scoliosis**. This deformity is found at birth or occurs early in life.

Pectus carinatum

Pectus carinatum is the anterior protrusion of the sternum and results in what is commonly called ***pigeon chest***. The deformity develops in childhood and in 50% of cases it occurs after the age of 10 years.

The **causes** of pectus excavatum and pectus carinatum are **unknown**. These disorders may run in families, so genetics may play a role. These conditions may be associated with connective tissue and metabolic disorders with excessive and defective growth of the costal cartilages, as in *Marfans Syndrome, Poland's Syndrome, Ehler Dunlos Syndrome, Noonan's Syndrome,* and *Homocystinurtia.*

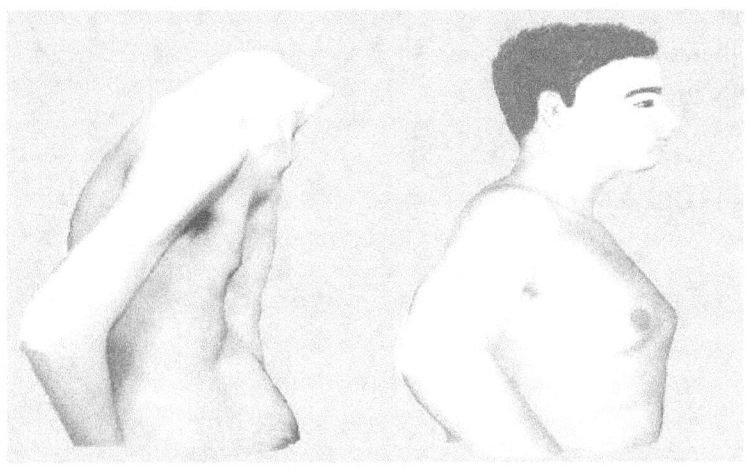

L   R

Figure: Pectus excavatum (L) and pectus carinatum(R)

Objective Questions (Set-5)

1. What occupies the pleural cavity?
2. Are the pleural cavities completely separated from each other?
3. Where is the parietal pleura separated from the visceral pleura?
4. Pleura develops from which germ layer?
5. What is the most dependant part of the pleural cavity in an ambulatory patient?
6. Through what areas is the needle passed during thoracocentesis?
7. What structures are encountered during thoracocentesis?
8. What is thoracocentesis?
9. Define pneumothorax.
10. Define pleural effusion.
11. Define chylothorax.
12. What is the blood supply and nerve supply of the pleura?

Multiple Choice Questions (Set-5)

1. Which of the following structures is NOT encountered by a needle during thoracocentesis at midaxillary line at the 6th intercostal space?
   A. External intercostal muscle
   B. Internal intercostal muscle
   C. Innermost intercostal muscle
   D. Levator costarum
   E. Parietal pleura

2. With a patient with pleural effusion in the standing position, fluid in the right pleural cavity tends to gravitate down to the:
   A. Horizontal fissure
   B. Oblique fissure
   C. Right costomediastinal recess
   D. Right costodiaphragmatic recess

3. Which pleura form the pulmonary ligament?
   A. Cervical pleura
   B. Mediastinal pleura
   C. Diaphragmatic pleura
   D. Costal pleura

MCQ (Set-5) Answers: 1. D; 2. D; 3.B

Movements of the thoracic wall

The principal function of the thoracic wall and the diaphragm is to alter the volume of the thorax and thereby move air in and out of the lungs. The dimensions of the thorax change in three different directions while breathing: vertical; lateral; and anteroposterior. The elevation and depression of the diaphragm significantly alter the vertical dimension of the thorax. The vertical length of the thorax increases when the muscle fibers of the diaphragm contract during **inspiration**. The vertical length of the thorax decreases when the diaphragmatic muscles relax during **expiration**. Changes in the anteroposterior and lateral dimensions result from elevation and depression of the ribs.

The anterior ends of the ribs are inferior to the posterior ends. When the ribs are elevated, they move the sternum upward and forward. When the ribs are depressed, the sternum moves downward and backward. This is called a *pump handle movement*. Pump handle movement changes the dimensions of the thorax in the anteroposterior direction. **The pump handle movement occurs when the upper ribs are elevated during inspiration.**

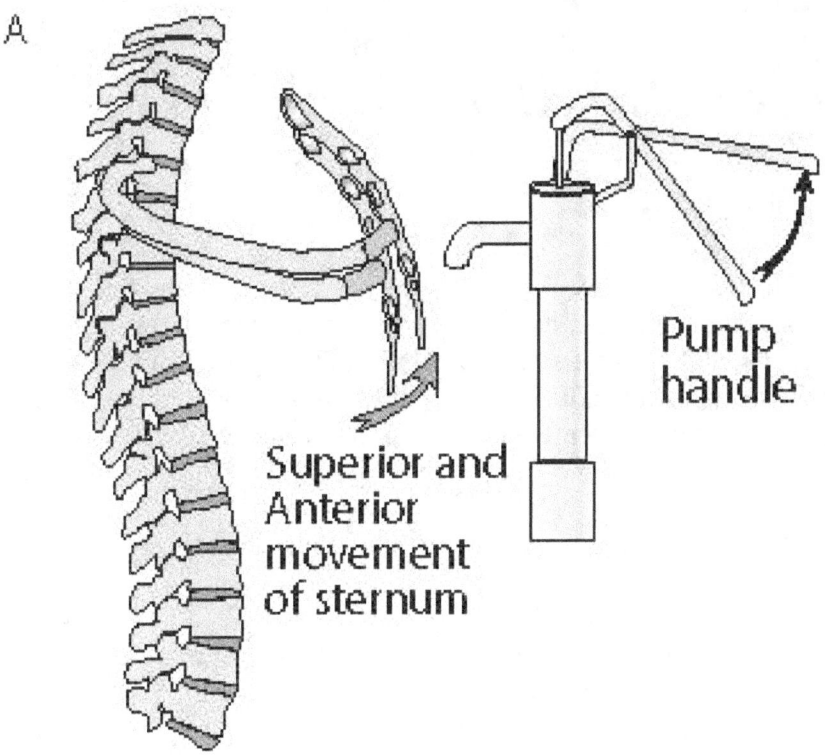

Figure: Pump handle movement

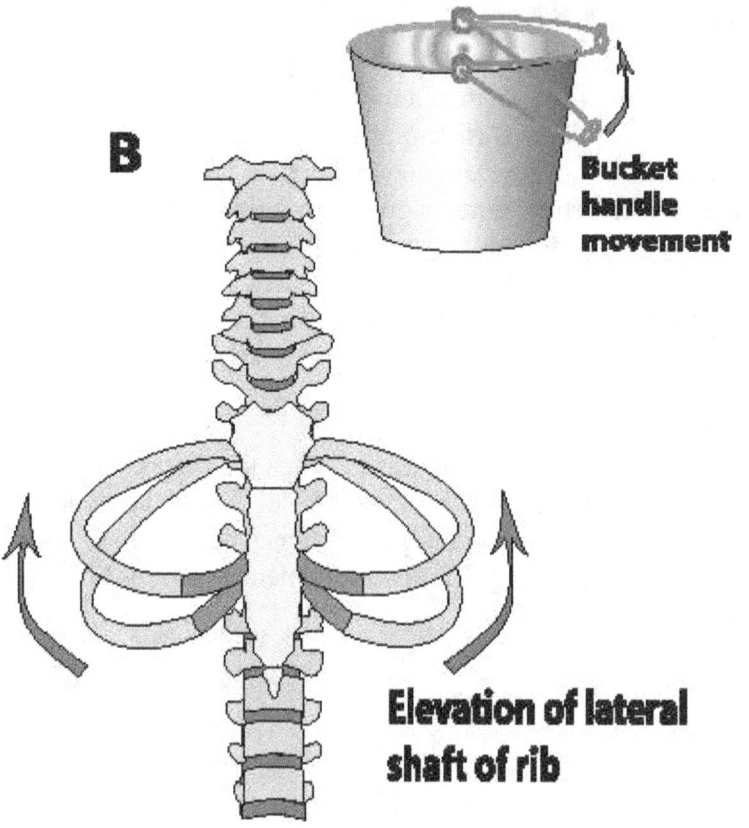

Figure: Bucket handle movement

Since the anterior ends of the ribs are lower than the posterior ends and the middles of the shaft tend to be lower than the two ends, when the shafts are elevated, the middle parts of the shafts move laterally. This creates a *bucket handle* movement. This bucket handle movement increases the lateral dimensions of the thorax. **Bucket handle movements are seen in the lower ribs during inspiration.**

Forced expiration involves contraction of the anterior abdominal muscles.

Slipping rib syndrome (dislocation of the rib)
Slipping rib syndrome is the displacement of a costal cartilage from the sternum. This condition is common in body contact sports. Complications of this syndrome are pressure on or damage to nearby nerves, vessels and muscles. Upon separation of the ribs or dislocation of the costochondral junction, the rib may move upward, overriding the rib above causing pain.

Paralysis of the diaphragm
Hemidiaphragm is paralysis of half of the diaphragm due to injury to its motor supply from the phrenic nerve. Because each half of the dome of the diaphragm has a separate nerve supply, only one side of the diaphragm is affected. In the past, purposeful dennervation to one side of the diaphragm was used as a management for Tuberculosis. In hemidiaphragm, there is paradoxical movement of the diaphragm, which can be seen in diagnostic images. During inspiration, the

paralyzed side moves upwards by the abdominal viscera and during expiration, the paralyzed side moves downward. These are opposite to the normal movement of the diaphragm which is undamaged.

Triangle of auscultation

Triangle of auscultation is located near the inferior border of the scapula and is bounded
superomedially by the inferolateral border of the trapezius, superolaterally by the rhomboid major, and inferiorly by the latissimus dorsi. The floor of the triangle of auscultation is formed by the **6th intercostal space**, and the 6th and 7th ribs. The floor is made distinct by folding the arms across the chest and flexing the trunk. This gap of triangle is a **good place** to examine the posterior segment of the lung with a stethoscope. The rib level of the superior angle of the scapula is the 2nd rib. The rib level of the inferior angle of the scapula is the 7th rib.

Breast/mammary gland

The breasts are two modified sweat glands present in both the sexes. The breast is rudimentary in males but well developed in female after puberty. It forms an important accessory organ of the female reproductive system and provides nutrition to the newborn in the form of milk.

Structure of the breast

The glandular part is composed of lobes , lactiferous ducts and forms parenchymal tissue. The stroma is partly fibrous and partly fatty. The lactiferous ducts have a dilatation near the nipple called *lactiferous sinus*. The lactiferous ducts are radially-arranged and reach the nipple. There are 16-20 lobes each with a lactiferous duct leading to lactiferous sinus then to the nipple. The lobes of the breast contain *tubuloalveolar* types of glands. Histologically, this is an example of *apocrine gland*. A part of the cell membrane is lost during the release of the secretion seen in lactating mothers. The *dermatome* over both the male and female nipples is T4. The nipple of the breast is a conical projection. The skin surrounding the base of the nipple is pigmented and forms a circular area called the *areola*. The areola is rich in modified sebaceous glands that become enlarged during pregnancy and lactation and forms a raised **tubercle of Montgomery**. Oily secretions from these glands lubricate the nipple and areola, and prevent the nipple from cracking during lactation. The parenchyma and stroma are more developed and vascular in a lactating breast.

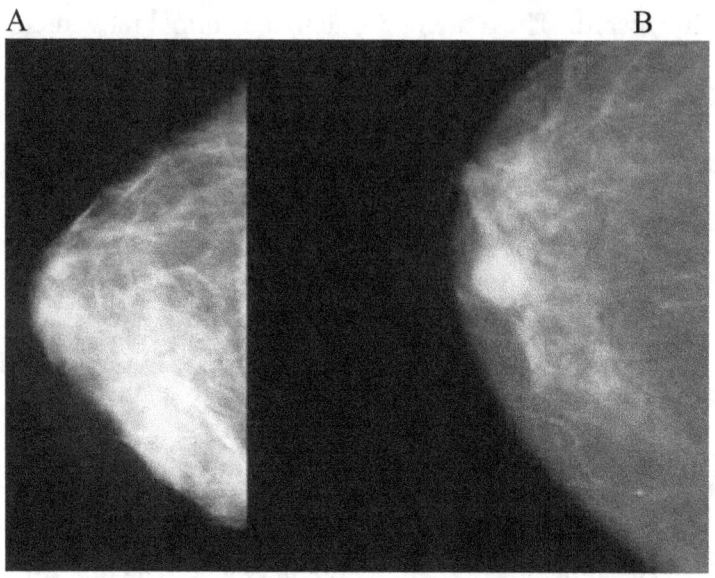

Figure of mammogram: A. Normal breast B. Cancer of the breast

Figure: Female breast

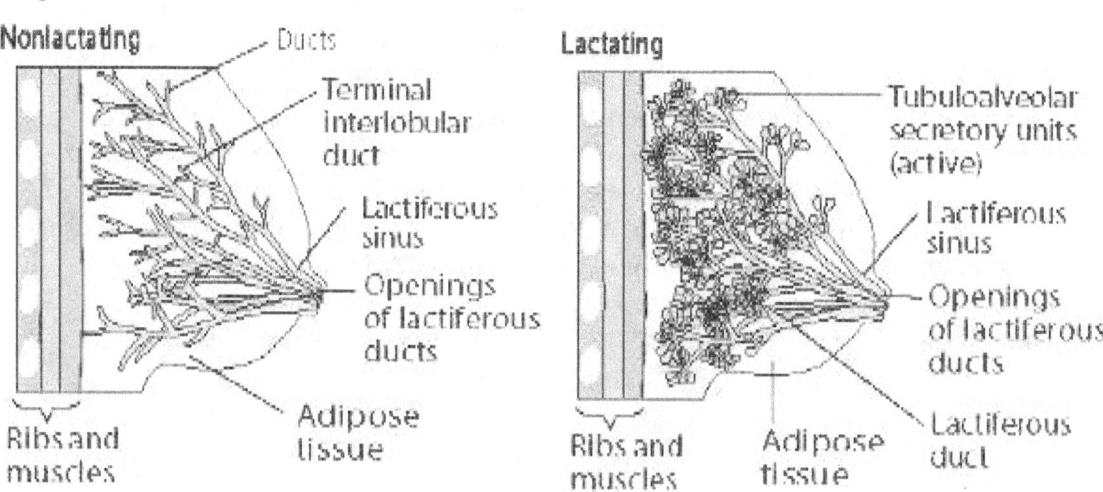

Location of the mammary gland

The breast lies in the superficial fascia of the pectoral region. A small extension of

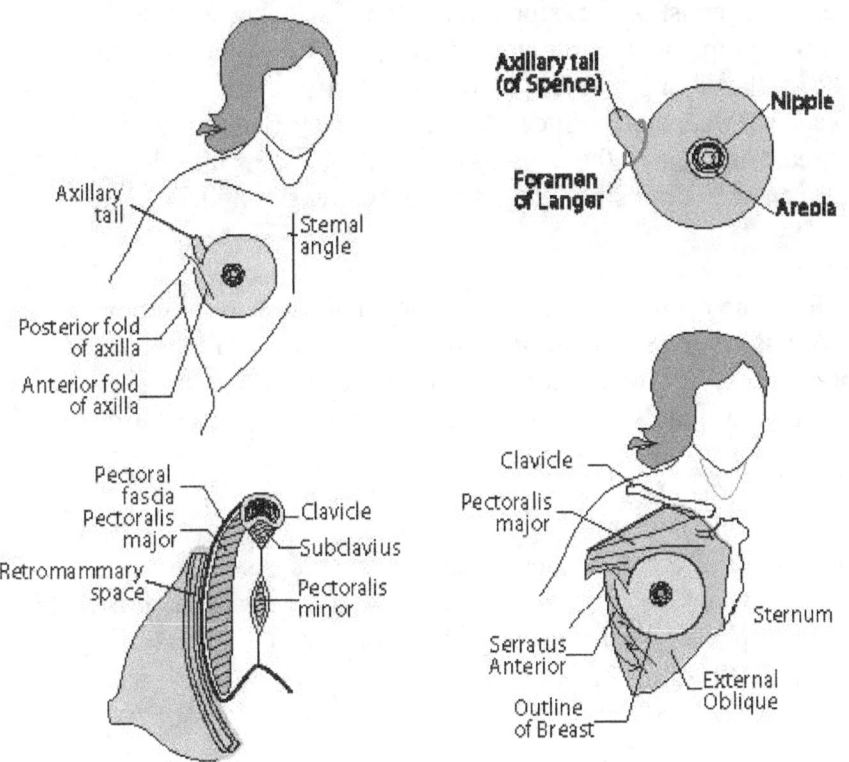

the mammary gland called the *axillary **tail of Spence*** is present in the inferolateral edge of the pectoralis major muscle. It pierces the deep fascia toward the axilla area (armpit). The breast extends vertically from the 2nd to 6th rib. Horizontally, it extends from the

Figure: Location and deep relations of the breast
Figure: Location and deep relations of the breast

lateral border of the sternum to the mid-axillary line. The nipple of the breast is in the **4th intercostal space** in the male and prepubertant girls. Nipple location is variable in adult women. The dermatome of the nipple is constant irrespective of age or sex and it is T4.

Muscles related to the breast and their nerve supply
The *pectoralis major* is innervated by lateral and medial pectoral nerves, which come from the lateral and medial cord of brachial plexus. *Pectoralis minor* lies beneath the pectoralis major and is not in direct contact with the breast. It is innervated by the medial pectoral nerve. *Serratus anterior* is innervated by the long thoracic nerve, which comes from the root of the brachial plexus C5, C6, and C7. The *external oblique* muscle is innervated by the lower intercostal nerves, which are also called the thoracoabdominal nerves.

Lymphatic drainage of the breast

The lymphatic drainage of the breast is very significant clinically because breast cancer can spread along the lymphatics to the regional lymph nodes. Lymph from the breast drains into the axillary lymph nodes, the parasternal (internal mammary) lymph nodes, and the posterior intercostal nodes. Approximately 75% of the lymph from the breast drains into the axillary nodes; 20% drains into the internal mammary nodes, and 5% drains into the posterior intercostal nodes.

Retromammary space

The breast is separated from the pectoral fascia by a loose areolar tissue called the *retro- mammary* space (bursa). The retromammary space contains a small amount of fat and allows the breast some degree of movement on the pectoral fascia. The spread of cancer cells to the retromammary space results in elevation of the entire breast.

Suspensory ligament (of Cooper)

The dermis of the breast is connected to the lactiferous duct by the suspensory ligament of the breast. The suspensory ligament of the breast is the condensation of the stromal tissue. The suspensory ligament provides support to the breast tissue.

Peau d´ orange sign (pig leather breast)

In breast cancer there is lymphatic obstruction and tightening of the suspensory ligament of the breast. It gives the skin a thickened, orange peel appearance called *Peau d´ orange sign.*

Mammography is the process of using low-dose amplitude-x-rays to examine the human breast and is used as a diagnostic and a screening tool. The goal of mammography is the early detection of breast cancer, typically through detection of characteristic masses and/or microcalcifications. Mammography is believed to reduce mortality from breast cancer.

Blood supply of the breast

The arterial supply of the breast is derived from the internal thoracic artery, a branch of the subclavian artery, through its perforating branches, the lateral thoracic, superior thoracic, and acromiothoracic branches of the axillary artery, and the lateral branches of the posterior intercostal arteries.

Nerve supply of the breast

The inferior and lateral cutaneous branches of the 4th to 6th intercostal nerves innervate the breast. The nerves do not control the secretion of the milk. Secretion is controlled by the hormone prolactin, secreted by the anterior pituitary gland.

Hormones acting on the breast

The overall growth of the breast is controlled by growth hormone, thyroid hormone, and corticosteroids. The ducts of the breast are developed by estrogen. The lobule and alveoli are developed by progesterone. The initiation of lactation is triggered by prolactin. The ejection of milk is done by the hormone oxytocin.

Development of the breast

The breast parenchyma (duct and lobule) develops from ectoderm. The stroma and fat develop from mesodermal tissue. The breast develops along the milk line also called **mammary ridge, or Line of Schultz.** The ridge extends from the axilla to the groin. In humans, the milk line disappears except in the pectoral region to develop one pair of mammary glands.

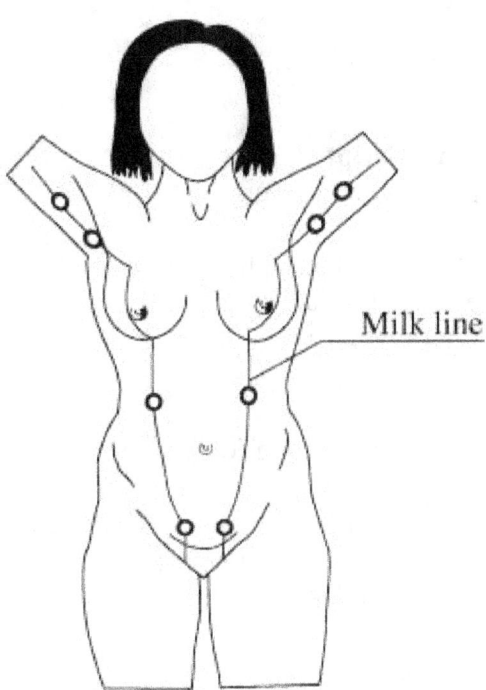

Milk line

Fig: Milk line with possible positions of accessory nipples

Congenital abnormality of the breast

The term polymastia is used to refer to the formation of multiple breasts. Polythelia is defined as multiple nipples. Amastia is development of no breasts.

Breast cancer in men

Approximately 1.5% of breast cancers occur in men. The **consequences are serious** because of late diagnosis and early metastasis. Carcinoma of breast affects approximately 1,000 men per year in the United States. A visible and palpable subareolar mass or secretion from a nipple may be the manifestation of the male breast cancer.

Gynecomastia

Gynecomastia is the **enlargement of the breast in males**. Gynecomastia is physiological in adolescent boys and may be associated with obesity. Drugs like furosemide, cimetidine, diethylstilbesterol, and digitalis may cause gynecomastia.Liver cirrhosis, liver cancer, or testicular cancer may be associated with gynecomastia. Gynecomastia is a symptom in 40% of Klinefelter's syndrome cases. Some types of testicular cancers are associated with gynecomastia.

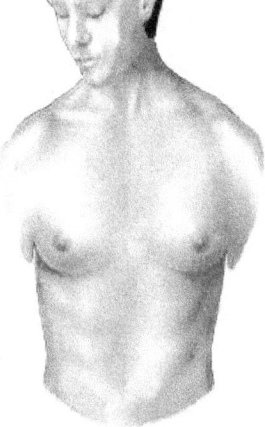

Figure: Gynecomastia

Objective Questions (Set-6)

1. Define pectus excavatum and pectus excarinatum.
2. What is slipping rib syndrome?
3. What are the boundaries of the triangle of auscultatioin?
4. What is the lymphatic drainage of the breast?
5. Which part or quadrant of the breast is mostly involved in breast cancer?
6. What is the blood supply of the breast?
7. What is Cooper's ligament?
8. What is the mechanism of peau d' orange or pigskin leather formation in breast cancer?
9. Why is there dimpling and or retraction of the nipple in breast cancer?
10. Why is there elevation of the entire breast seen in breast cancer?
11. What is the location of the mammary glands and nipple in relation to the ribs and axillary lines?
12. What is the function of gland of Montgomery?
13. What is Gynecomastia? What are the causes of gynecomastia?
14. What is the incidence of breast cancer in males in the US? What is the clinical importance of breast cancer in males?
15. What is the location of the nipple in males?

Multiple Choice Questions (Set-6)

1. Which of the following muscles does NOT form the boundary of the triangle of auscultation?
   A. Latissimus dorsi
   B. Terse major
   C. Rhomboid major
   D. Trapezium

2. Which of the following quadrants/sites is the most common site of breast cancer?
   A. Upper and outer quadrant
   B. Upper and inner quadrant
   C. Lower and outer quadrant
   D. Lower and inner quadrant
   E. Nipple and areola

3. Lymph from the breast drains mostly to which of the following groups of lymph nodes?
   A. Parasternal lymph nodes
   B. Subphrenic lymph nodes
   C. Lateral thoracic lymph nodes
   D. Axillary lymph nodes

4. Which of the following hormones stimulate the growth of ducts of the breast?
   A. Estrogen
   B. Progesterone
   C. Oxytocin
   D. Prolactin

5. Select an INCORRECT statement:
   A. Breasts develop from the endoderm.
   B. Breasts are located on the 2nd to 6th ribs.
   C. Areola of the breast is hairless.
   D. Skin of the areola has sebaceous glands.
   E. The breast extends from the parasternal line to the midaxillary line.

MCQ (Set-6) Answers: 1. B; 2. A; 3. D; 4. A; 5. A

Poland syndrome

Poland syndrome has multiple anomalies including the absence of both the pectoralis major and pectoralis minor muscles. Poland syndrome also includes the deficiency of two to four ribs, maldevelopment of the breast, lower positioning of the breast and anomalies in the fingers.

Intercostal nerves

The intercostal nerves are the anterior primary rami of thoracic spinal nerves 1 through 11. The first and second intercostal nerves also innervate the upper limb. The spinal segments T3-T6 supply only the thoracic wall hence are called typical intercostal nerves. The lower five intercostal nerves (T7-T11) also supply the abdominal walls and are called thoracoabdominal nerves. The anterior primary rami of the 12th thoracic nerve form the subcostal nerve. Dorsal primary rami of the spinal nerves innervate the erector spinae. Intercostal nerves and vessels pass through the internal intercostal and innermost intercostal muscles. Gray and white rami communicans connect the sympathetic trunk to the intercostal nerves. The intercostal nerves move along **a posterior to anterior course along the length of each intercostals space**.

Because nerve plexus formation does not occur in relationship to the thoracic wall, the pattern of **peripheral and segmental (dermatomal) innervations is identical in both the sides.**

Intercostobrachial nerve

Intercostobrachial nerve is the lateral cutaneous branch of T2. This nerve is linked with *referred pain* from the medial aspect of the upper extremity in the *Ischemic Heart Diseases.*

Cold abscess

Cold abscess is a localized collection of pus, which may develop in the body of the thoracic vertebra and extend through the route of the intercostal nerves. Cold abscess is a feature of **tuberculosis**.

Herpes Zoster

Herpes Zoster is the dormant virus of chicken pox (varicella zoster) flare-ups and causes blistering along the intercostal nerves, especially along the **lateral and anterior** cutaneous branches. Herpes zoster or Shingles is associated with severe chest pain. Herpes Zoster may affect the **ophthalmic division of trigeminal** nerve or the facial nerve. The virus may remain dormant in the dorsal root ganglion, trigeminal ganglion or geniculate ganglion for many years. Herpes zoster is seen when the immunity of a person is decreased as in cancer, old age, or any other debilitating condition. It may involve one or two dermatomes unilaterally depending on the virulence of the virus. Involvement of the facial nerve may cause **Ramsay Hunt syndrome** with facial paralysis, deafness, unilateral loss of taste and skin lesion around the ear. Shingles may, on occasion, involve the genitals or upper leg. Involvement of the ophthalmic nerve may lead to **corneal ulcer and blindness**.

Objective Questions (Set-7)
1. What is Poland Syndrome?
2. What is the importance of intercostobrachial nerve?
3. What nerves may be involved in herpes zoster?

Multiple Choice Questions (Set-7)
1. Select an INCORRECT statement about the herpes zoster:
   A. Herpes zoster is caused by a bacteria
   B. Herpes zoster blisters are seen along the cutaneous branches of an intercostal nerve
   C. Herpes zoster develops when the immunity is low in debilitating conditions like cancer
   D. Herpes zoster may involve ophthalmic nerve
   E. Herpes zoster may involve geniculate ganglion

2. Which of the following branches of the internal thoracic artery supply the breast?
   A. Musculophrenic artery
   B. Pericardiacophrenic artery
   C. Superior epigastric artery
   D. Perforating branches of the internal thoracic artery

MCQ (Set-7) Answers: 1. A; 2. D

Intercostal arteries

Each intercostal space contains one posterior intercostal artery with its collateral branch, and two anterior intercostal arteries. The **greater part** of the intercostal space is supplied by the posterior intercostal artery.

Posterior intercostal arteries

There are eleven pairs of intercostal arteries. The **first** and **second** posterior intercostal arteries arise from the **superior intercostal artery** which is a branch of the costocervical branch. The **third to eleven** posterior intercostal arteries arise from the **descending thoracic aorta.**

Anterior intercostal arteries

There are nine *intercostal spaces* anteriorly and there are two intercostal arteries in each intercostal space. In the upper six spaces, the anterior intercostal arteries are branches from the **internal thoracic artery.** In intercostal spaces seven through nine, the arteries are branches of the musculophrenic artery.

The anterior and posterior intercostal arteries and veins **anastomose** in approximately the **anterior axillary line.**

Internal thoracic artery

The *internal thoracic artery* arises from the first part of the subclavian artery. It has the following branches:

- Pericardiacophrenic artery (**accompanies the phrenic nerve**)
- Mediastinal arteries
- **Two** anterior intercostal arteries in the upper six intercostal spaces
- Perforating branches (large in lactating breast)
- Superior epigastric artery*
- Musculophrenic artery*

> ****The internal thoracic artery terminates at 6th intercostal space lateral to the sternum into 1. Superior intercostal artery and 2. Musculophrenic artery.**

Azygos vein (azygos means unpaired)

The *azygos vein* drains the posterior thoracic wall and the upper lumbar region. It forms an important channel **connecting** the superior and inferior vena cava. The azygos vein is formed by the union of the right subcostal vein and right ascending lumbar vein opposite vertebra **L1 or L2.** The azygos vein enters the thorax by passing through the **aortic opening** of the diaphragm. The azygos vein ascends up to the level of T4, where it arches forward over the root of the right lung, and **ends in the superior vena cava.**

Tributaries of the azygos vein

1. Right superior intercostal vein (formed by the union of the 2nd, 3rd and 4th posterior intercostal veins)
2. Hemiazygos vein

3. Accessory hemiazygos vein
4. Right bronchial vein
5. Several esophageal, mediastinal,vertebral, and pericardial veins
6. Fifth to eighth right posterior intercostal veins

Notes

The *superior vena cava* is formed by the union of the left and right brachiocephalic veins.

- Left *brachiocephalic vein* is longer than the right brachiocephalic vein.
- Azygos vein receives hemiazygos and accessory hemiazygos veins.
- Hemiazygos vein receives blood from the upper left posterior chest wall.
- Accessory hemiazygos vein receives blood from the lower left posterior chest wall.

Sympathetic trunks

The *ganglionated chains* are located one on each side of the vertebral column. They extends from the base of the skull to the coccyx. Usually, there are ten to eleven pairs of sympathetic ganglia present in the thoracic region. In total, twenty-two to twenty-five ganglia are present in the sympathetic trunk. There are only three cervical sympathetic ganglions (superior, middle and intermediate). *Stellate* **or** *Cervicothoracic ganglion* is formed by the fusion of the last cervical ganglion and the first thoracic ganglion. The stellate ganglion is located in front of the transverse process of the T7 vertebra. The sympathetic trunk is connected to the intercostal nerves by the gray and white **rami communicans**. The lower end of the sympathetic trunk unites in front of the coccyx in a ganglion called *ganglion impar*.

Vagal trunks

The anterior and posterior *vagal trunks* are derived from the *esophageal plexus*. The esophageal plexus is formed by the **left and right** *vagus nerves* **and sympathetic nerves** from the sympathetic trunk and the greater splanchnic nerve. The vagal trunks enter the abdomen through the esophageal opening of the diaphragm.

Splanchnic Nerves

The medial branches of the lower seven sympathetic ganglia form the splanchnic nerves. The ***greater splanchnic nerve*** is formed by five roots ganglia T5 to T10. It pierces the *crus of the diaphragm* and ends in the celiac ganglion, aorticorenal ganglion and in the suprarenal gland.

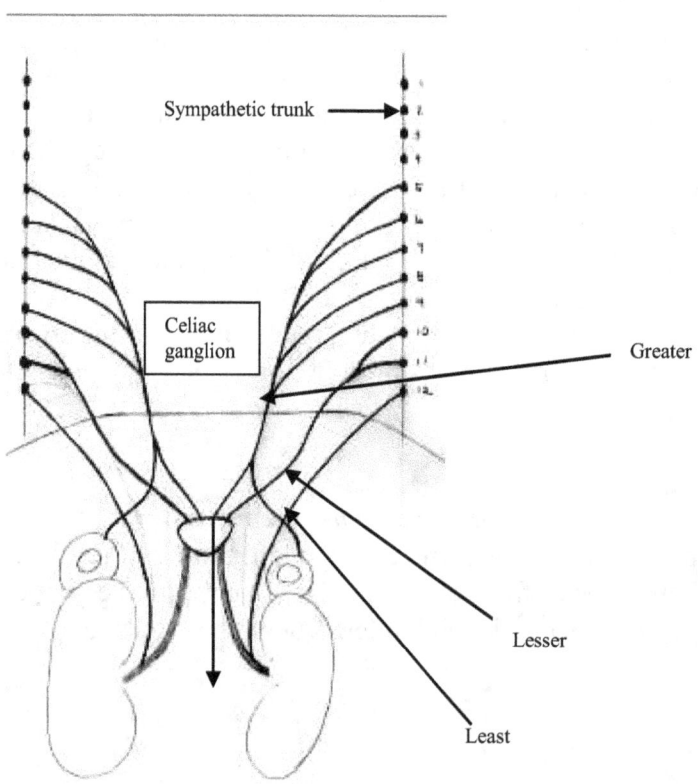

Figure: Sympathetic trunk and splanchnic nerves

The *lesser splanchnic nerve* is formed by two roots from ganglia ten and eleven. It pierces the crus of the diaphragm and ends in the celiac ganglion.
The *least splanchnic nerve* is tiny and often absent. It arises from one root from ganglion twelve and ends in the renal ganglion.

The **celiac ganglion** is the same as the **solar ganglion**. This ganglion is located around the celiac trunk. The splanchnic nerves contain preganglionic sympathetic fibers. These preganglionic fibers synapse in the *prevertebral ganglia* like celiac ganglion (plexus), aortic plexus, or renal plexuses.

Structures piercing the clavipectoral fascia
1. Cephalic vein
2. Thoracoacromial artery
3. Lateral pectoral nerve
4. A few lymph vessels

Notes
- Fluid accumulates first in the costodiaphragmatic recesseses in pleural effusion.

Route of a pulmonary embolism
An *embolus* is usually formed in the calf muscles like the soleus, in the varicose veins, or in the pelvic veins. The route that the embolism follows once it reaches the inferior vena cava is through the right atrium, the right ventricle, and the pulmonary trunk, ending in the pulmonary arteries. A pulmonary embolism is caused by prolonged immobilization like a long plane flight or recovery after surgery. It can also arise from the effects of estrogen in the oral contraceptive pill in women over the age of thirty-five, and with a history of smoking.

Features of Klinefelters Syndrome (47XXY genotype)
Klinefelters Syndrome is a male phenotype generally affecting tall, thin, and lean individuals causing azospermia and male sterility. Barr body is present and in 40% of cases has associated gynecomastia.

Costochondritis (Tietzes Syndrome)
Costochondritis is a condition commonly seen in twenty to forty year old females. There is pain in the sternochondral joint. The cause is unknown, but may be associated with trauma or road traffic accident.

Objective Questions (Set-8)
1. What are the branches of the internal thoracic artery?

2. How many intercostal arteries are present in the anterior and posterior intercostal spaces?
3. The posterior intercostal arteries are branches of which arteries?
4. The anterior intercostal arteries are branches of which arteries?
5. What is the route of pulmonary embolism?
6. What are the features of Klinefelters Syndrome?
7. What are the dermatomes of a male and female breast nipple, clavicle, and xiphoid process?
8. What is Tietzes Syndrome?
9. Which artery accompanies the phrenic nerve?

Multiple Choice Questions (Set-8)
1. The chicken pox virus may remain dormant in which of the following parts of the nervous system before manifesting as Shingles.
   A. Anterior gray horn
   B. Posterior gray horn
   C. Lateral gray horn
   D. Dorsal root ganglion
   E. Gray rami communicans

2. Which of the following arteries is NOT a branch of the internal thoracic artery?
   A. Musculophrenic artery
   B. Lateral thoracic artery
   C. Superior epigastric artery
   D. Pericardiacophrenic artery
   E. Anterior intercostal artery

3. Which of the following structures passes in between the scalene anterior and scalene medius?
   A. Subclavian artery
   B. Subclavian vein
   C. Vertebral artery
   D. Common carotid artery
   E. External carotid artery

4. The anterior and posterior intercostal arteries anastomose approximate at the_____.

   A. Anterior axillary line
   B. Midaxillary line
   C. Posterior axillary line
   D. Parasternal line
   E. Paravertebral line

MCQ (Set-8) Answers: 1. D; 2. B; 3. A; 4. A

Nerves of the thorax

Nerve	Origin	Course	Innervation	Clinical notes
Phrenic Nerve	• Ventral rami of C3-C5 nerves • Phrenic nerve contains both motor and sensoryfibers	Passes over the scalene anterior muscle, superior thoracic aperture, superior media-stinum, middle mediastinum, reaches the diaphragm, and gall bladder	• Diaphragm, Mediastinal pleura • Gall bladder • Fibrous and parietal layers of serous pericardium • Diaphragmatic pleura • Diaphragmatic peritoneum	• Paralysis in one side may cause hemidiaphragm • Characterized by paradoxical movement of the diaphragm • Referred pain to the shoulder in cholelithiasis, basal pneumonia, and in pleural effusion
Vagus Nerve	Medulla of brainstem	Passes as a content of the carotid sheath, superior mediastinum, posterior mediastinum, and continues to the abdomen through the esophageal opening of the diaphragm as anterior and posterior vagal trunks.	• Pulmonary plexus • Cardiac plexus • Esophageal plexus	• Vagotomy is done to decrease the secretion of acid in the stomach • Vagus nerve may be damaged at the brainstem, or it may be lacerated in the neck region • Characterized by deviation of the uvula and soft palate; hoarseness of voice
Recurrent laryngeal nerves	Vagus nerve	The right recurrent laryngeal nerve goes around the right subclavian artery. The left recurrent laryngeal nerve runs around the arch of aorta. Both the nerves ascend along the tracheoesophageal groove.	• All the intrinsic muscles of the larynx • Except cricothyroid (external laryngeal nerve • Sensory innervation to the larynx inferior to the level of the vocal cord	• Lesion in the recurrent laryngeal nerve causes hoarseness of voice • Involvement of the nerves by the carcinoma or itatrogenic damage in thyroidectomy
Esophageal plexus	• Vagus nerve • Sympathetic ganglia • Greater splanchnic nerve	Located on the middle and lower third of the esophagus. Forms the anterior and posterior vagal trunks that reaches the abdomen through the	• Parasympathetic and sympathetic innervations to the esophagus	

		esophageal opening of the diaphragm		
Pulmonary plexus	• Vagus nerve • sympathetic trunk	Forms at the root of the lungs and is distributed along the bronchial subdivisions	• Parasympathetic fibers (vagal) are bronchoconstrictors • Increase bronchial secretions • Sympathetic (T2-T5) fibers are bronchodilators	
Cardiac Plexus	• Vagus nerve • Sympathetic trunk (cervical and upper thoracic sympathetic ganglia)	The superficial cardiac plexus is situated below the arch of the aorta and in front of the right pulmonary artery. The deep cardiac plexus is situated in front of the bifurcation of the trachea and behind the arch of the aorta	• Parasympathetic fibers (vagal) decrease heart rate. • Sympathetic fibers increase the heart rate	
Intercostal nerves	Ventral rami of T1-T11 nerves	Pass between the innermost intercostal and internal intercostal muscles along the intercostal spaces and costal grooves	• Innervates the muscles • skin of the intercostal spaces • Lower 7 nerves innervate the skin and muscles of the abdomen	
Subcostal nerve	Ventral ramus of T12 nerve	Passes along the inferior border of the 12th rib and reaches the lower abdominal wall	• Skin of the lower abdomen • Lateral side of the gluteal region • Lower parts of the abdominal wall muscles (obliques and transverse abdominis) • Pyramidalis muscle • Peritoneum	

Notes
- Sympathetic nerves arise from the lateral horns of the L1 to L2 segments of the spinal cord.
- Nerve supply to muscles is motor (associated with muscle contraction with movements).
- Nerve supply to skin and peritoneum is sensory (associated with sensations like pain, touch, and temperature).

Objective Questions (Set-9)
1. What is the root value of the phrenic nerve?
2. What is the course of the phrenic nerve in the middle mediastinum?
3. What structures are innervated by the phrenic nerve?
4. What is a hemidiaphragm?
5. What is the course of the left recurrent laryngeal nerve?
6. What types of fibers are present in the phrenic nerve?

Multiple Choice Questions (Set-9)
1. An **INCORRECT** statement about the phrenic nerve is that it
   .
   A. passes over the scalene medius.
   B. innervates mediastinal pleura.
   C. innervates diaphragmatic pleura.
   D. innervates fibrous and parietal pericardium.

2. Which of the following nerves hooks around the arch of the aorta, passes close to the ligamentum arteriosum and ascends between the trachea and esophagus to the larynx?
   A. Left phrenic nerve
   B. Left recurrent laryngeal nerve
   C. Right vagus nerve
   D. Right recurrent laryngeal nerve
   E. Right phrenic nerve

3. During an open heart surgery a surgeon gives longitudinal incision on the fibrous pericardium in lieu of a transverse incision in order to save the:
   A. Vagus nerve
   B. Phrenic nerve
   C. Hemiazygos vein
   D. Azygos vein
   E. Internal thoracic artery

4. The pain from an inflamed gall bladder may be referred to the right supraclavicular region. The referred pain from the inflamed gall bladder is carried by the:
   A. right vagus nerve
   B. right phrenic nerve
   C. right recurrent laryngeal nerve
   D. right greater splanchnic nerve

5. Which of the following arteries accompanies the phrenic nerve?
   A. Internal thoracic artery
   B. Musculophrenic artery
   C. Pericardiacophrenic artery
   D. Superior epigastric artery

MCQ Answers (Set-9): 1. A; 2. B; 3. B; 4. B 5. C

Joints of the thorax

Joints	Type	Articulation	Ligaments	Notes
Manubriosternal joint (also called sternal angle or angle of Louis)	Secondary cartilaginous joint (symphysis) May be a synostosis above the age of 30	Articulation between the manubrium and the body of the sternum (mesosternum)	Fibrous membrane. (May be connected by bone called synostosis)	Permits slight movement during respiration
Costovertebral	Plane type of synovial joint	With the upper costal facet of corresponding vertebra and the inferior costal facet of the vertebra superior to it	Radiate and intra-articular ligaments of the head of the rib Capsular ligament	
Costotransverse	Plane type of synovial joint	The tubercle of a typical rib articulates with the transverse process of the corresponding vertebra	Capsular ligament and costotransverse ligaments	Upper costotransverse joints permit pump-handle movement and the lower costotransverse joints permit bucket-handle movement
Costochondral	Primary cartilaginous joint	Joint between the anterior end of the rib and the lateral end of the costal cartilage	Periosteum connects the bone and the cartilage	
Sternocostal or chondrosternal	First sternocostal joint is a primary cartilaginous joint. Second to seventh sternocostal joints are synovial joint of plane variety.	Articulates the medial ends of the costal cartilages (1st to 7th) to the lateral border of the sternum		
Interchondral	Synovial joint of plane variety	Articulations between 6th and 7th, 7th and 8th, and 8th and 9th costal cartilages	Interchondral ligaments	The joint between 9th and 10th costal cartilages is fibrous type
Sternoclavicular	Saddle type of synovial joint	Articulation between the medial end of the clavicle, the clavicular notch of the manubrium, and 1st costal cartilage	Anterior and posterior sternoclavicular ligaments, and interclavicular ligament	Associated with the movement of the shoulder girdle
Xiphisternal	Primary cartilaginous	Articulation between the		

	joint. May be a synostosis in older individuals	xiphoid process and the body of the sternum		
Intervertebral	Secondary cartilaginous joint(symphysis)	Joint between the adjacent vertebral bodies	Anterior and posterior longitudinal ligaments, ligamenta flava, interspinous and supraspinous ligaments, interspinous and intertransverse ligaments	Vertebrae act together to allow flexion, extention, lateral bending and rotation

Notes
- Synostosis is the union between bones by small pieces of bones.

Objective Questions (Set-10)
1. Classify the joints of the thorax
2. Give an example of a primary cartilaginous and a secondary cartilaginous joint
3. Name the plane synovial joints in the thorax
4. Name the ligaments related to the intervertebral disc.

Multiple Choice Questions (Set-10)
1. Which of the following joints is a secondary cartilaginous joint?
   A. Sternoclavicular joint
   B. Interchondral joint
   C. Costochondral joint
   D. Manubriosternal joint
   E. Costotransverse joint

2. Which of the following veins connects the superior and inferior vena cava?
   A. Azygos vein
   B. Internal thoracic vein
   C. Right brachiocephalic vein
   D. Right subclavian vein

MCQ (Set-10) Answers: 1. D; 2. A

Veins of the thoracic wall

Name of the vein	Location of the vein	Tributaries of the vein	Drain into	Notes
Superior Vena Cava	1st right costal cartilage to the third right costal cartilage near the sternum	Azygos vein, small veins of the pericardium and mediastinal structures, left and right brachiocephalic veins	Right atrium of the heart. Drains blood from the upper part of the body above the level of the diaphragm	There may be two superior vena cava. Superior vena cava obstruction is a feature of mediastinal syndrome. There may be left superior vena cava which opens into the coronary sinus
Right brachiocephalic vein	The right brachicephalic vein extends from the medial end of the right clavicle to lower border of the 1st right costal cartilage	Right vertebral vein, right internal thoracic vein, right inferior thyroid vein	Unites with the left brachiocephalic vein to form the superior vena cava	Right brachiocephalic vein is shorter than the left brachiocephalic vein
Left brachiocephalic vein	The left brachiocephalic vein extends from posterior to the medial end of the left clavicle to the right 1st costal cartilage	Left vertebral vein, left internal thoracic vein, superior intercostal vein, left inferior thyroid vein sometimes 1st left posterior intercostal vein, thymic and pericardial veins	Unites with the right brachiocephalic vein to form the superior vena cava	Left brachiocephalic vein is longer than right brachiocephalic vein (6 cm vs 2cm).
Azygos vein	Formed in the abdomen, enters the thoracic cavity through the aortic opening of the diaphragm at the level of T12, extends along the right anterolateral surface of the thoracic vertebral column up to the T4 vertebra	Hemiazygos vein, accessory hemiazygos vein, right superior intercostal vein, 5th to 11th right posterior intercostal veins, right bronchial vein, esophageal veins, pericardial veins, mediastinal veins, right ascending lumbar vein and right subcostal vein	Drains into the superior vena cava	Azygos vein is the connecting channel between the superior and inferior vena cava. If the superior vena cava is obstructed the blood may reach to the right atrium through the inferior vena cava
Hemiazygos vein	Formed in the abdomen, pierces the left crus of the diaphragm, and	9th, 10th and 11th left posterior intercostal veins, left ascending lumbar vein, left	Drains into the azygos vein	

	extends left anterolateral surface of the thoracic vertebral column between T12 to T8	subcostal vein, esophageal veins and mediastinal veins		
Accessory hemiazygos vein	Drains venous blood from 4th to 8th left intercostal spaces and descends to the upper left anterolateral surface of the thoracic vertebral column (T4-T8)	4th to 8th left posterior intercostal veins, and sometimes left bronchial vein	Drains into the azygos vein. Sometimes hemiazygos and accessory hemiazygos veins unite together and forms a common channel that opens into the azygos vein	
Inferior vena cava	Formed in the abdomen in front of righr anterolateral surface of the L5, enters the thorax through the vena caval opening at the central tendon of the diaphragm. It has a very short course in the thorax	There is **no** tributary of the thoracic part of the inferior vena cava	Opens at the right inferolateral aspect of the right atrium	Thoracic part of the inferior vena cava is very short and lies within the pericardial cavity
Left superior intercostal vein	Left anteraolateral surface of the thoracic vertebral column. Drains blood from the 2nd, 3rd and 4th intercostal spaces	Left 2nd, 3rd and 4th posterior intercostal veins, left bronchial vein usually and sometimes left pericardiacophrenic vein	Opens into the left brachiocephalic vein	
Right superior intercostal vein	Right anterolateral surface of the thoracic vertebral column	Right 2nd, 3rd and 4th posterior intercostal veins	Opens into the azygos vein	
Posterior intercostal veins (eleven pairs)	One posterior intercostal vein in each intercostal space	Veins from the vertebral canal, vertebral venous plexus, and the veins from the muscles and skin of	1st left intercostal vein opens into the left brachiocephalic vein.	

		the back drains into the posterior intercostal vein	1st right intercostal vein opens into the right brachiocephalic vein. 2nd, 3rd, and 4th right posterior intercostal vein opens into the right superior intercostal vein. 2nd, 3rd, and 4th left posterior intercostal veins open into the left superior intercostal vein. 5th to 11th right posterior intercostal vein and subcostal vein open azygos vein. 5th to 8th left posterior intercostal vein opens into the accessory hemiazygos vein. 9th to 11th left posterior intercostal veins and left subcostal vein open into the hemiazygos vein	
Esophageal veins (numerous)	Present throughout the length of the esophagus	Submucosal venous plexus and periesophageal venous plexus	Thoracic esophageal veins are tributaries of azygos vein, hemiazygos vein, accessory hemiazygos vein and intercostal veins	Esophagus is a site of porto-caval anastomosis. Submucosal venous plexus is enlarged to form esophageal varices in case of portal hypertension e.g., cirrhosis of liver or liver cancer. Esophageal varices may rupture and may cause hematemesis.

Anterior intercostal veins(9 pairs)	Each upper nine intercostal spaces has two anterior intercostal arteries each		1st to 6th anterior intercostal veins open into the internal thoracic veins. 7th to 9th anterior intercostal veins open into the musculophrenic vein	Anterior intercostal veins anastomose with the posterior intercostal veins
Internal thoracic vein	Passes along the parasternal border accompanying the internal thoracic artery anterior to the sternalis muscle	Anterior intercostal veins of the upper six intercostal spaces, and pericardiacophrenic veins	Opens into the brachiocephalic vein	
Thoracoepigastric vein	Located in the superficial fascia of the lateral surface of the abdomen and thorax. This vein connects the superficial epigastric vein (atributary of femoral vein) to the lateral thoracic vein (a tributary of the axillary vein)	Unnamed tributaries in the lateral wall of the thorax and abdomen	Opens above to the lateral thoracic vein. Opens below to the superficial epigastric vein	In vena caval obstructions, the thoracoepigastric vein opens up, connecting the great sapheneous vein to the axillary vein

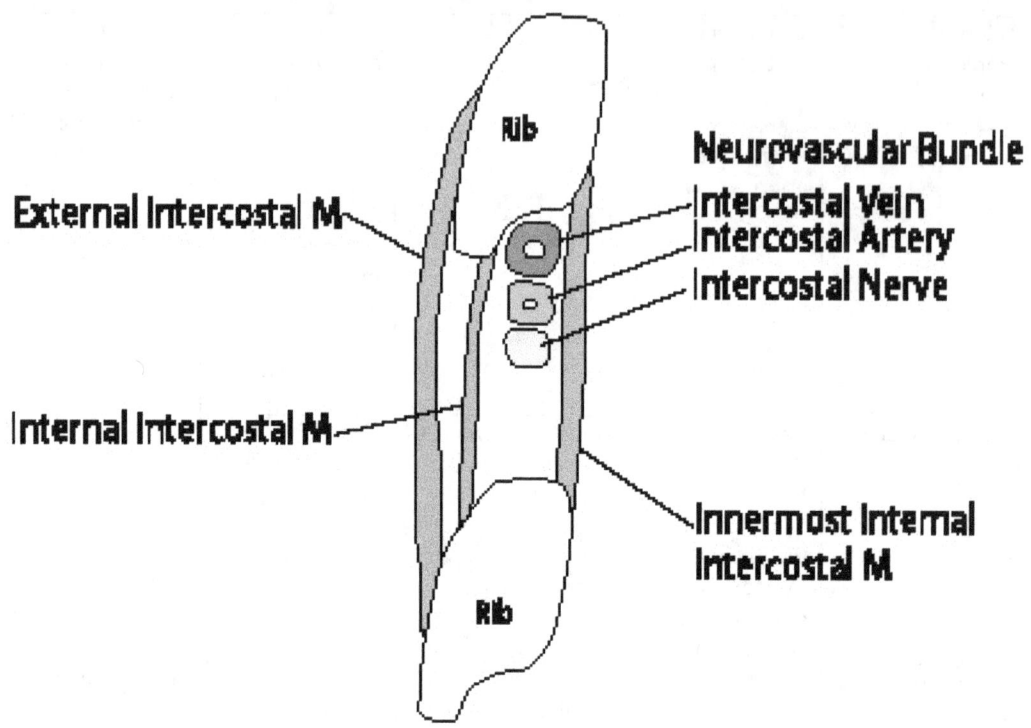

Figure: Neurovascular bundle in a typical intercostal space

Objective Questions (Set-11)
1. How is the superior vena cava formed?
2. Which two veins join to form the left brachiocephalic vein?
3. How is the azygos vein formed and where does it terminate?
4. What are the tributaries of the azygos vein?

Multiple Choice Questions (Set-11)
1. Which of the following veins connects the superior and inferior vena cava?
   A. Azygos vein
   B. Internal thoracic vein
   C. Right brachiocephalic vein
   D. Right subclavian vein

2. Which of the following veins has no valve?
   A. Azygos vein
   B. Hemiazygos vein
   C. Accessory hemiazygos vein
   D. Subclavian vein
   E. Superior vena cava

3. Azygos vein opens into which of the following veins?
   A. Hemiazygos
   B. Accessory hemiazygos vein
   C. Inferior vena cava
   D. Superior vena cave
   E. Right superior intercostal vein

4. Right superior intercostal vein is a tributary of the:
   A. Superior vena cava
   B. Inferior vena cava
   C. Azygos vein
   D. Hemiazygos vein
   E. Accessory hemiazygos vein

MCQ (Set-11) Answers: 1. A; 2. E; 3. D; 4. C

Arteries of the thoracic wall

Name of artery	Location	Branches	Supply to	Clinical notes
Descending thoracic aorta	Begins from the end of the arch of the aorta and ends as the abdominal aorta. Located on the left side of the thoracic vertebral column in the posterior mediastinum extending from T4 to T12	Nine posterior (3rd to 11th) intercostal arteries, subcostal artery on each side, esophageal arteries, two left bronchial arteries, pericardial arteries, mediastinal arteries, superior phrenic arteries	Posterior thoracic wall, structures of the mediastinum (e.g., esophagus, pericardium), bronchi, the diaphragm, and the spinal cord	Descending thoracic aorta is a site of dissecting aneurysm (abnormal dilatation of the blood vessel)
Internal thoracic artery	Originates from the subclavian artery (2 cm above the sternal end of the clavicle) to its termination at the 6th intercostal space, descends vertically behind the 1st six costal cartilages approx 1cm from the lateral sternal border	1 Anterior intercostal arteries, 2. Musculophrenic, 3. Pericardiacophrenic 4. Superior epigastric artery, 5. Mediastinal arteries, 6. Perforating arteries	Anterior thoracic wall, mediastinum and breast	Internal thoracic artery is often used in CABG (Coronary Artery Bypass Grafting)
Anterior intercostal arteries (9 pairs)	1st to 6th is branches of the internal thoracic artery. Seventh to ninth anterior intercostal arteries are branches of the musculophrenic artery. Located in the 1st to 9th anterior intercostal spaces in between internal intercostal and innermost intercostal muscles	Muscular and cutaneous branches	Intercostal muscles, skin and parietal pleura	There are two anterior intercostal arteries in each intercostal space. One coursing above and one coursing below the rib.
Posterior intercostal arteries (11 pairs)	1st and 2nd posterior intercostal arteries are branches of superior intercostal artery. 3rd to 11th posterior inter-costal arteries are branches of descending thoracic aorta	Dorsal, collateral, muscular, radicular and cutaneous branches	Muscles , skin of the back and meninges of the spinal cord	There is one posterior inter-costals artery in each intercostal space. Posterior and anterior intercostal arteries anastomose freely
Subcostal artery	Descending thoracic aorta.	Dorsal, collateral, muscular, radicular,	Muscles of the anterolateral	Subcostal artery accompanies

	Passes along the inferior order of the 12th rib	and cutaneous branches	abdominal muscles and skin of the back,	subcostal nerve
Lateral thoracic artery	Arises from the 2nd part of the axillary artery, passes along the lateral border of the pectoralis minor then deep to the pectoralis major upro the 5th intercostal space	Muscular branches, and lateral mammary branches, and cutaneous branches	Pectoralis major and minor, serratus anterior, subscapularis, axillary lymph nodes , and skin	**This artery passes over the serratus anterior muscle (usually the artery passes beneath the muscle)
Thoracoacromial artery	Arises from 2nd part of the axillary artery. A short artery lies along the medial border of the pectoralis minor and then pierces the clavipectoral fascia	Acromial, pectoral, clavicular, and deltoid branches	Muscles (pectoralis major and minor, deltoid and subclavius and sternoclavicular joint	Pierces the clavipectoral fascia *Clavipectoral fascia is a fibrous sheet between the pectoralis minor and subclavius muscles and lies deep to the clavicular part of the pectoralis major
Ascending aorta	Arises from the left ventricle; passes behind the manubrium sterni	1.Left coronary artery 2. Right coronary artery	Wall of the heart including the conductive system of the heart	
Arch of the aorta	Continues from ascending aorta to the descending thoracic aorta behind the manubrium sterni and in front of the trachea	1. Brachiocephalic trunk 2. Left common carotid artery 3. Left subclavian artery	1. Upper extremity 2. Head and Neck 3. Brain	*Aneurysm of the arch of the aorta may cause difficulty in breathing (dyspnea) and swallowing (dysphagia) due to compression on the trachea or esophagus.
Brachio-cephalic trunk	First branch of the arch of aorta. Located behind the right side of the manubrium sterni	1. Right common carotid artery 2. Right subclavian artery	1. Right side of the head and neck 2. Right upper extremity	*The right recurrent laryngeal nerve hooks around the right subclavian artery and ascends to the tracheoesophageal groove

Notes

- **<u>Three blood vessels may be used in CABG (Coronary Artery Bypass Grafting). Theses are the internal thoracic artery, the great saphenous vein and the radial artery.</u>**
- The right posterior intercostal arteries are longer than the left posterior intercostal arteries because the aorta is on the left side and the right has to cross over the backbone.

Musculophrenic artery

The *Musculophrenic artery* runs downwards and laterally behind the 7th, 8th, and 9th costal cartilages. The musculophrenic artery gives two anterior intercostal bracnches to each of these three spaces. It pierces the diaphragm near the 9th costal cartilage and terminates on the undersurface of the diaphragm.

Superior epigastric artery

The *superior epigastric artery* passes downwards behind the 7th costal cartilage and enters the rectus sheath by passing between the costal and sternal slips of the diaphragm. In the rectus sheath it passes longitudinally downwards behind the rectus abdominis muscle to anastomose with the inferior epigastric artery at the level of the umbilicus.

Aneurysm

Aneurysm means abnormal dilation of the blood vessel. Aortic aneurysm may be associated with congenital bicuspid valve, atherosclerosis, Marfan syndrome, and Ehlers Danlos Syndrome etc.

Dysphagia lusoria

Dysphagia lusoria is diffculty in swallowing due to entanglement of the esophagus by the aberrant vessels.

Highest intercostal artery

Highest intercostal artery is a branch of the costocervical trunk. The first and second posterior intercostal arteries are the branches of the highest intercostal arteries.

Objective Questions (Set-12)

1. From what vertebral level does the descending thoracic aorta begin and end?
2. What structures are supplied by the descending thoracic aorta?
3. What is the site of termination of the internal thoracic artery?
4. What are the courses, area of distributions and terminations of the superior epigastric artery and musculophrenic artery?
5. What is the first branch of the arch of the aorta?
6. What is the clinical importance of the internal thoracic artery?
7. What are the branches of the brachiocephalic trunk?
8. What structure is hooked around by the right recurrent laryngeal nerve?

Multiple Choice Questions (Set-12)

1. Which of the following artery is a branch of the brachiocephalic trunk?
   A. Internal thoracic artery
   B. Musculophrenic artery
   C. Pericardiacophrenic artery
   D. Right subclavian artery
2. Superior epigastric artery is a branch of the_____.
   A. musculophrenic artery
   B. pericardiacophrenic artery

C. internal thoracic artery

D. internal iliac artery

MCQ (Set-12) Answers: 1. D; 2. C

Muscles of the thoracic wall

Muscle	Origin	Insertion	Nerve supply	Action
External intercostal (11 pairs)	Inferior border of the upper rib of a intercostal space	Superior border of the lower rib of a intercostal space	Intercostal nerves (T1-T11)	Elevate the ribs in inspiration
Internal intercostal (11 pairs)	Floor of a costal groove and adjacent costal cartilage of the upper rib of an intercostal space	Upper border of the rib below	Intercostal nerves (T1-T11)	Act on the ribs in expiration (in active or forced respiration)
Innermost intercostal, located deep to the internal intercostal, well-developed in the middle 2/3rd of lower intercostal spaces	Same as internal intercostal	Same as internal intercostal	Adjacent intercostal nerves	Acts along with internal intercostal
Levator costarum (12 pairs)	Tranverse process of C7 to T11	Between the tubercle and angle of the rib below	Intercostal nerves	Elevates the rib in respiration
Serratus posterior superior	Lower part of the nuchal ligament and spinous process of the upper thoracic vertebrae	Upper borders of the 2nd to 5th ribs	Intercostal nerves (T2-T5)	Elevates the ribs. Its role in man is uncertain
Serratus posterior inferior	Spinous process of the T11, T12, L1, L2, and L3 with their supraspinous ligament	Outer border of the T9, T10, T11, and T12 lateral to their angles	Ventral rami of the 9th, 10th, 11th and 12th thoracic spinal nerves	Depresses the rib
Transversus thoracis	Posterior surface of the body of the sternum and the xiphoid process	2nd to 6th costal cartilages	Intercostal nerves (T2-T6)	Depresses the ribs
Subcostals (well developed only in the lower part of the thorax)	Internal surface of one rib near its angle	Internal surface of one or two rib below	Lower intercostal nerves	Depresses the rib

Notes

- There are three scaleni muscles: anterior, middle, and posterior.
- Scalene muscles take origin from the transverse process of the cervical vertebrae.
- Scalenus anterior and medius are inserted to the 1st rib.
- Scalenus posterior inserts on the 2nd rib.
- Scalenus minimus is an extension of the scaleneus anterior.

Extrinsic muscles covering the thorax

Muscle	Origin	Insertion	Nerve Supply	Action
Pectoralis major	1. Anterior surface of the medial half of the clavicle 2. Anterior surface of the sternum 3. Upper six costal cartilages 4. Aponeurosis of the external oblique muscle	Lateral lip of the intertubercular sulcus	Medial and lateral pectoral nerves	1. Adduction and medial rotation of the shoulder 2. Flexion of the arm (by clavical head 3. Sternocostal head extends it form the flexed position and also helps in climbing
Pectoralis minor	3rd-5th ribs near costochondral junction	Medial border and upper surface of the coracoid process of scapula	Medial pectoral nerve	1. Draws the scapula anteriorly 2. Depresses the point of the shoulder 3. Helps in forced inspiration
Serratus Anterior	Outer surfaces of the lateral part of the upper 8 ribs	Costal surface of medial border of the scapula	Long thoracic nerve	Protraction and rotation of the scapula. Keeps the medial border and of scapula opposed to the thoracic wall
Latissimus dorsi	1. Posterior $1/3^{rd}$ of the iliac crest. 2. Thoracolumbar fascia. 3. Spinous process of T7-T12. 4. 9th-12th ribs. 5. Inferior angle of the scapula	Floor of the intertubercular sulcus of the humerus	Thoracodorsal nerve (**C6,C7**,C8)	1. Adducts, extends, and rotates humerus medially. 2. Raises body toward arms during climbing
Trapezius	1. Medial $1/3^{rd}$ of the superior nuchal line 2. External occipital protuberance 3. Ligamentum nuchae 4. C7-T12 spinous processes	1. Posterior border or lateral $1/3^{rd}$ of the clavicle 2. Medial margin of the acromion 3. Spine of the scapula	1. Spinal accessory nerve (CN XI, motor) 2. C3 and C4 nerves (Pain and Proprioception)	1. Upper fibers elevate the scapula as in shrugging 2. Middle fibers retracts the scapula 3. Rotates the scapula 4. Steadies the scapula
Levator scapulae	Transverse processes of C1-C4	Medial border of the scapula superior to root	1. Dorsal scapular nerve (C5) 2. Cervical	Raises scapula

		of the spine	nerves (C3, C4)	
Rhomboid major	Spinous processes of 2nd to 5th thoracic vertebrae	Medial border of the scapula from the level of the spinous process of the scapula to the inferior angle	Dorsal scapular nerve (C4, C5)	Retract and fixes scapula
Rhomboid minor	1. Ligamentum nuchae 2. Spinous process of C7 and T1	Smooth triangular area at the medial end of the spine of the scapula	Dorsal scapular nerve (C4, C5)	Retract and fixes the scapula
Subclavius	Junction of the 1st rib and its costal cartilage	Undersurface of the middle third of the clavicle	Nerve to the subclavius (C5, C6)	Depresses lateral end of the clavicle
Rectus abdominis	Pubic crest and symphysis pubis	Xiphoid process, 5th, 6th, and 7th costal cartilages	T7 to T11 intercostal nerves and subcostal nerves	1. Flexes the trunk 2. Supports abdomen
External oblique	External surface of the 5th -12th rib	Iliac crest, pubic tubercle, and linea alba	T7 to T11 intercostal nerves and subcostal nerves	Flexes , rotates vertebral column, compress abdominal viscera

Erector spinae muscle

Erector spinae muscle is also called sacrospinalis. As the name implies, the muscle originates from the sacrum and inserts on the spinous of the lumbar, the 11th and 12th thoracic vertebrae and iliac crest, which then splits and inserts as the *Iliocostalis*, *Longissimus* and *Spinalis*. **Mnemonic: I Love Spine**. Iliocostalis has three subdivisions: the lumborum; thoracis; and cervicis. Longissimus has three subdivisions: the thoracis; cervicis; and capitis. Spinalis has three subdivisions: the thoracis; cervicis; and capitis. Erector spinae is innervated by posterior rami of spinal nerves. **The actions of erector** spinae are two-fold: acting bilaterally it extends the vertebral column; acting unilaterally it laterally flexes the vertebral column.

Transversospinalis muscle

Transversospinalis muscle has three subdivisions: *Semispinalis*; *Multifidus*; and *Rotatores*. Semispinalis has three divisions: thoracis, cervicis, and capitis. Rotatores muscle is best developed in the thoracic region. The action of Transversospinalis muscle is mainly to extend and stabilize the vertebral column. The nerve supply is the posterior rami of spinal nerves.

Objective Questions (Set-13)
1. What are the parts of the erector spinae muscle?
2. What is the innervation of the erector spinae muscle?
3. What are the actions of the erector spinae?
4. What are the components of the Transversospinalis muscle?
5. Which muscle is the deepest subdivision of the transversospinalis muscle?

Multiple Choice Questions (Set-13)
1. Which of the following muscles is absent in Poland Syndrome?
   A. Latissimus dorsi
   B. Trapezius
   C. Serratus posterior superior
   D. Serratus posterior inferior
   E. Pectoralis major

2. Winged scapula is caused by paralysis of which of the following muscles?
   A. Pectoralis major
   B. Pectoralis minor
   C. Serratus anterior
   D. Serratus posterior superior
   E. Serratus posterior inferior

MCQ (Set-13) Answers: 1. E; 2. C

Pericardium

The pericardium is a fibroserous membrane that covers the heart and the beginning/end of the great vessels close to the heart. The pericardium develops from **mesoderm**. The pericardium is a closed sac and is located in the **middle mediastinum.** The tough external layer is called the **fibrous pericardium**, fuses superiorly to the tunica adventitia of great vessels and inferiorly with the **central tendon** of the diaphragm. The inner surface of the fibrous pericardium is lined with a shiny serous membrane called the parietal layer of serous pericardium. The parietal layer of serous pericardium is reflected onto the heart at the great vessels (aorta, pulmonary trunk, pulmonary veins, superior vena cava and inferior vena cava) as the visceral layer of serous pericardium. The visceral layer of serous pericardium over the heart forms the **epicardium**. The serous pericardium is composed of mainly of **mesothelium**, a single layer of flattened cells forming an epithelium that lines both the internal surface of the fibrous pericardium and the outer surface of the heart.

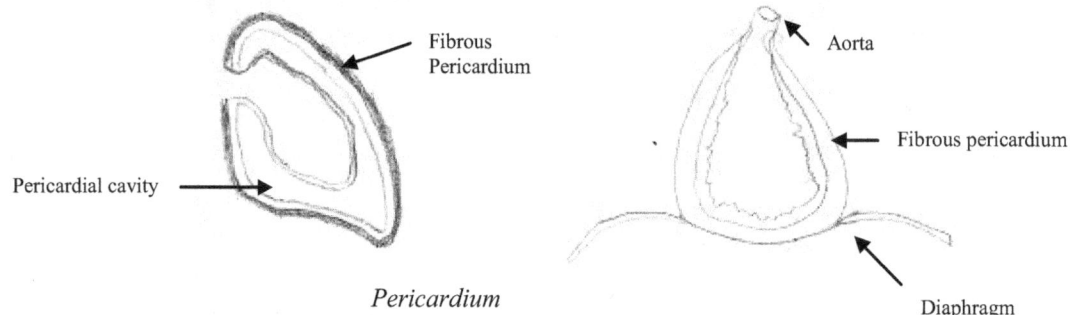

Pericardium

The fibrous pericardium is composed of **collagen fibers** and has little ability to distend acutely. Anteriorly the fibrous pericardium is connected to the posterior aspects upper and lower parts of the body of the sternum by the weak superior and inferior sternopericardial ligament.

The **phrenic nerve and the pericardiacophrenic artery** descend through the superior and middle mediastinum. These structures pass over the lateral aspect of the fibrous pericardium and are vulnerable to injury during open heart surgery. The thoracic segment of the **inferior vena cava** is very short, lies within the pericardial cavity. Therefore to expose this portion of the inferior vena cava, the pericardial sac must be opened.

Pericardial cavity

The pericardial cavity contains 1. Heart with cardiac vessels 2. Ascending aorta 3. Pulmonary trunk 4.Lower half of the superior vena cava 5. Terminal part of the inferior vena cava and the 6. The terminal parts of pulmonary veins. The *pericardiacophrenic ligament* is the site of continuity between the inferior wall of the fibrous pericardium and the central tendon of the diaphragm. The cavity is a potential space between opposing layers of the parietal and visceral layers of the serous pericardium. It normally contains a thin film of fluid(<20ml.) that enables the heart to move and beat in a frictionless environment. There are two pericardial sinuses called the *transverse sinus* and the *oblique sinus*.

The *transverse pericardial sinus* sinus is a transverse gap between the arterial and venous end of the heart tube. It is bounded anteriorly by the ascending aorta and pulmonary trunk, posteriorly by the superior vena cava, and inferiorly by the left atrium. On each side it opens into the general pericardial cavity. This sinus is utilized by the cardiac surgeons to pass a finger or ligature from one side of the heart to the other.

The *oblique pericardial sinus* is a narrow gap behind the heart. It is bounded anteriorly by the left atrium (hence posterior to the base of the heart), and posteriorly by the pericardium. Below and left it opens into the pericardial cavity. It is a cul-de-sac, acting as a potential space for left atrial systole and diastole.

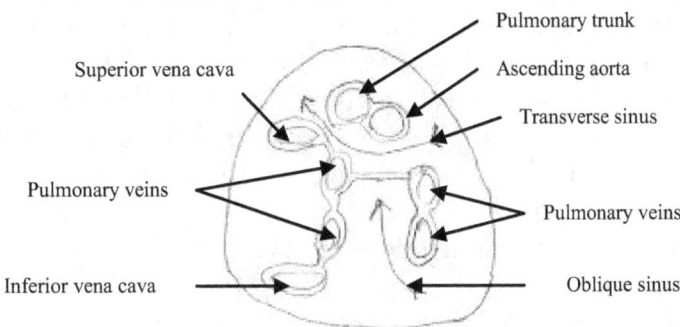

Transverse and Oblique Sinus

Arterial supply of the pericardium
Multiple arteries supply the fibrous pericardium and parietal layer of serous pericardium. The arteries are branches from internal thoracic artery, pericardiacophrenic artery, the musculophrenic artery, bronchial arteries, esophageal arteries, superior phrenic arteries and branches of descending thoracic aorta. The visceral layer of the serous pericardium (epicardium) is supplied by the coronary arteries.

Venous drainage of the pericardium
The venous drainage of the pericardium is through the internal thoracic vein, pericardiacophrenic vein, and the tributaries of azygos vein.

Nerve supply of the pericardium
The phrenic nerve (C3-C5) innervates the fibrous pericardium and parietal layer of serous pericardium. This is the primary source of sensory fibers. Pain sensation conveyed by these nerve fibers is commonly referred to the C3-C5 dermatomes. The epicardium (visceral layer of the serous pericardium) is innervated by vagus nerve (parasympathetic). The sympathetic fibers to the fibrous and serous pericardium is vasomotor.

Clinical notes on pericardium
- *Pericarditis* is an inflammatory condition of the pericardium. The common causes of pericarditis are viral infection, bacterial infection, systemic illness (such as chronic renal failure) and post myocardial infarction. Symptom includes chronic central chest pain which may radiate to the shoulder. Pain from pericarditis may be relieved by sitting forward in a tripod position.

Pericardial friction rub may be auscultated due to friction between the rough parietal and visceral layer of the serous pericardium.

- *Pericardial effusion* is a collection of fluid in the pericardial cavity, which can be clear or purulent.
- *Cardiac Tamponade (heart compression)* is a **rapid** accumulation of excess fluid within the pericardial sac which compresses the heart. Cardiac tamponade may occur after trauma, proximal extension from a dissecting aortic aneurysm or cardiac surgery. The fibrous pericardium is relatively fixed structure that cannot expand rapidly. There is quick accumulation of fluid in the pericardial cavity that compresses the right atria, superior and inferior vena cava and results in heart failure due to lack of venous return. The **right atrium is compressed first because of its thin wall.** The veins of the face and neck become engorged because of the backup of the blood. Clinical finding includes hypotension (blood pressure [BP] 90/40 mm of Hg) that does not respond to rehydration. Cardiac tamponade can rapidly progress to cardiogenic shock and death.
- Collection of blood in the pericardial sac (e.g., in stab wound) is called *hemopericardium*.
- *Pericardiocentesis* is the removal of fluid from the pericardial cavity. Pericardiocentesis is a procedure to relieve cardiac tamponade or pericardial effusion. This can be done by inserting a wide-bore needle through the left 5th or 6th intercostal space near the lateral sternal border. This approach protects the left pleura and lung. The pericardial sac may also be reached by entering the left costoxiphoid angle, located between the left margin of the xiphoid process and the costal margin, and passing the needle superolaterally.

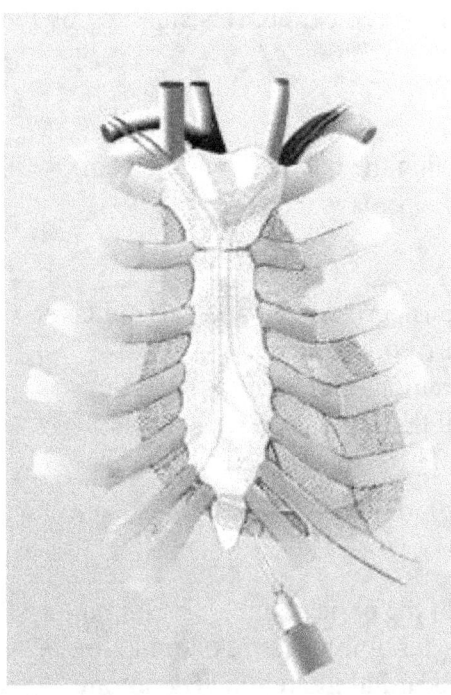

Figure: Pericardiocentesis through subxiphoid approach

Structures penetrated by the sternal approach of the pericardiocentesis
1. Skin 2. Superficial fascia 3. Pectoralis major muscle 4. External intercostals muscle 5. Internal intercostals muscle 6. Transverse thorasis muscle 7. Fibrous pericardium and 8. Parietal layer of serous pericardium.
**The internal thoracic artery, branches of the coronary arteries, and pleura may be damaged during this maneuver.

Structures penetrated by the subxiphoid approach of pericardiocentesis
1. Skin 2. Superficial fascia 3. Anterior rectus sheath 4. Rectus abdominis muscle 5. Transverse abdominis muscle 6. Fibrous pericardium and 7. Parietal layer of seous pericardium
**The central tendon of the diaphragm and the left lobe of the liver may be damaged during this maneuver.

Objective Questions (Set-14)
1. What is fibrous pericardium?
2. What is serous pericardium?
3. Define hemopericardium and cardiac tamponede.
4. Why is engorgement of face and neck veins seen in cardiac tamponade?
5. What is pericardial effusion?
6. What is the difference between pericardial effusion and cardiac tamponade?
7. How is pericardiocentesis performed?
8. What is epicardium? What is the blood supply and nerve supply of the epicardium?
9. What vessels accompany the phrenic nerve?
10. What is the boundary of the transverse pericardial sinus and what is its clinical importance?
11. What is the boundary of the oblique pericardial sinus and what is its clinical importance?
12. What are the contents of the pericardial cavity?

Multiple Choice Questions (Set-14)
1. The parietal layer of serous pericardium is lined by_____.
   A. simple squamous epithelium
   B. stratified squamous epithelium
   C. transitional epithelium
   D. simple columnar epithelium
   E. simple cuboidal epithelium

2. Structurally the fibrous pericardium is composed of_____.
   A. cardiac muscle
   B. collagen fibers
   C. cartilage
   D. bone

3. Select an incorrect statement
    A. The visceral layer of the serous pericardium is lined by simple squamous epithelium.
    B. The visceral layer of the serous pericardium is also called epicardium.
    C. The epicardium is supplied by the coronary arteries.
    D. The epicardium is innervated by the phrenic nerve.

4. Which of the following arteries accompanies the phrenic nerve?
    A. Superior epigastric artery
    B. Musculophrenic artery
    C. Internal Thoracic artery
    D. Pericardiacophrenic artery

MCQ (Set-14) Answers: 1. A; 2.B; 3.D, 4.D

Lungs

The lungs are the vital organs of respiration. The main function is to oxygenate the blood by bringing inspired air into close relation with the venous blood in the pulmonary capillaries. The lungs are separated from each other by the mediastinum to which they are attached by the root of the lungs.

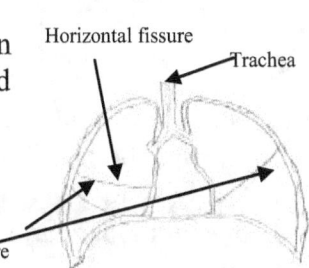

Lungs and pleura

Fissures of the lungs

The fissures of the lung divide each lung into lobes. The right lung has two fissures: the oblique fissure and the horizontal or transverse fissure. The *oblique fissure* lies parallel to a line interconnecting the T4 spinous process posteriorly, the 5th rib in the midaxillary line and the 6th costal cartilage anteriorly. It separates the superior and middle lobe from the inferior lobe in the right lung; it also separates the superior from the inferior lobe in the left lung. The *horizontal fissure* passes from the oblique fissure from the 5th rib in the midaxillary line laterally to the 4th costal cartilage anteriorly.**The horizontal fissure may or may not touch the anterior border of the right lung**.The horizontal fissure separates the superior lobe from the middle lobe in the right lung. It is absent in the left lung.

The left lung has one fissure: the oblique fissure. All the fissures of the lung are covered by the visceral pleura.The fissures reach the hilum. The number of fissures and lobes in the lungs may vary. Sometimes a fissure may be incomplete.

Roots of the lung

The root of the lung is a short, broad pedicle which connects the medial surface of the lung to the mediastinum. It is formed by the structures which either enter or exit the lung at hilum. The root of each lung lies opposite the bodies of T5, T6 and T7.

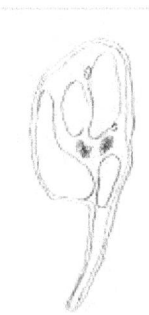

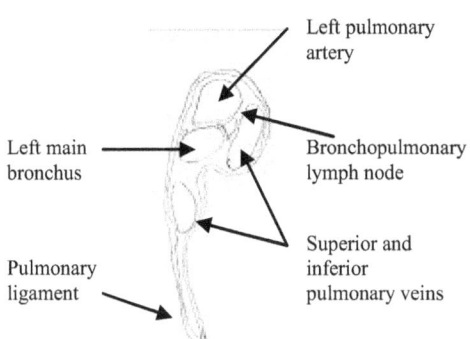

Right root of lung *Left root of lung*

Contents of the root of the lung
- Principal bronchus on the left side, eparterial and hyparterial bronchi on the right side.
- One pulmonary artery
- Two pulmonary veins, superior and inferior
- Bronchial arteries, one on the right side and two on the left side
- Bronchial veins
- Anterior and posterior pulmonary plexus of nerves
- Lymphatics of the lung
- Bronchopulmonary lymph nodes
- Aveolar tissue

Arrangement of structures in the root of the lung
Anterior to posterior
1. Superior pulmonary vein
2. Pulmonary artery
3. Bronchus

Superior to inferior
Right side
1. Eparterial bronchus
2. Pulmonary artery
3. Hyparterial bronchus
4. Inferior pulmonary vein
Left side
1. Pulmonary artery
2. Bronchus
3. Inferior pulmonary vein

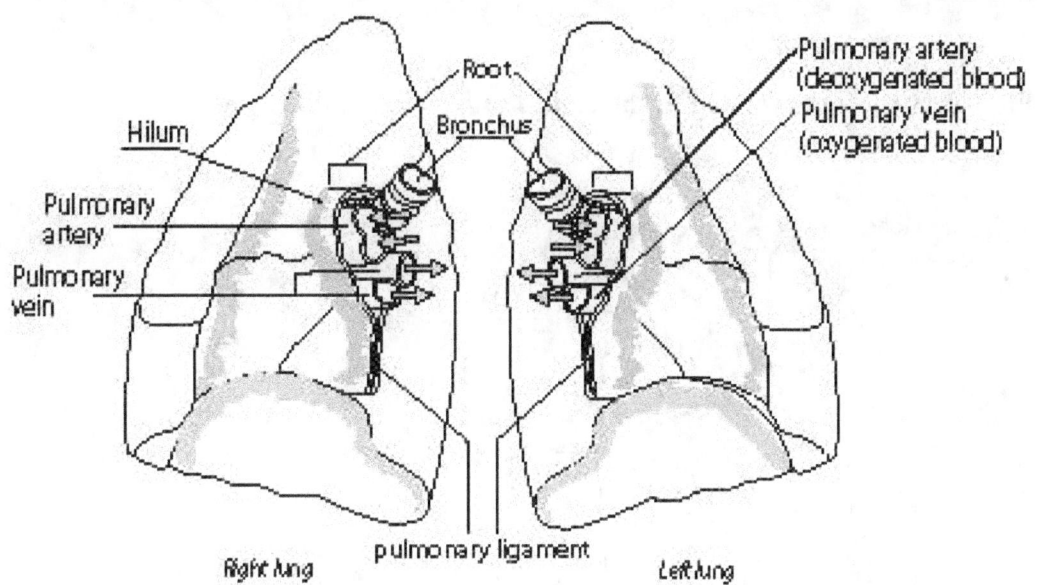

Hilum

Root

Bronchus

Pulmonary artery
(deoxygenated blood)

Pulmonary vein
(oxygenated blood)

Pulmonary
artery

Pulmonary
vein

pulmonary ligament

Right lung

Left lung

Figure: Structures related to the right lung

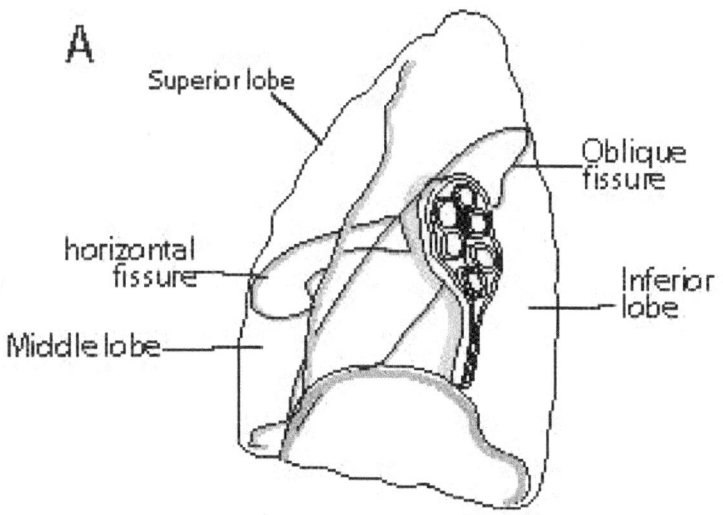

A
Superior lobe
Oblique fissure
horizontal fissure
Middle lobe
Inferior lobe

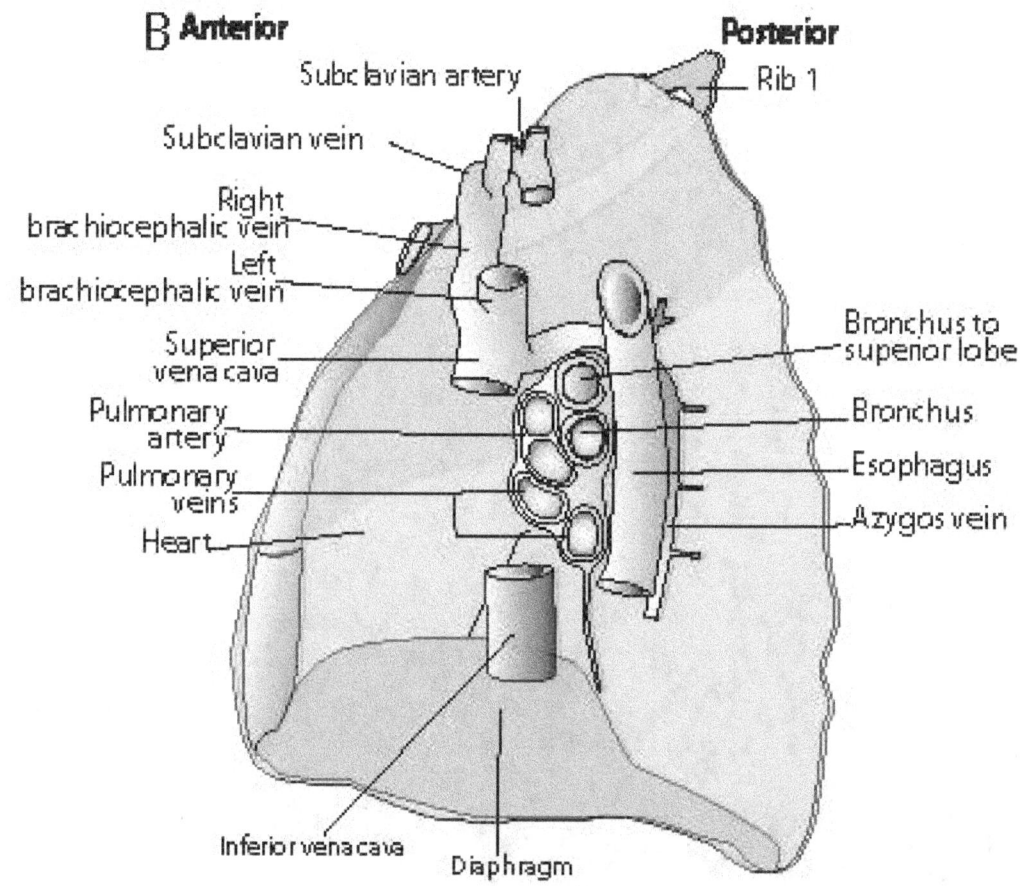

B Anterior

Posterior

Subclavian artery

Rib 1

Subclavian vein

Right brachiocephalic vein

Left brachiocephalic vein

Superior vena cava

Pulmonary artery

Pulmonary veins

Heart

Bronchus to superior lobe

Bronchus

Esophagus

Azygos vein

Inferior vena cava

Diaphragm

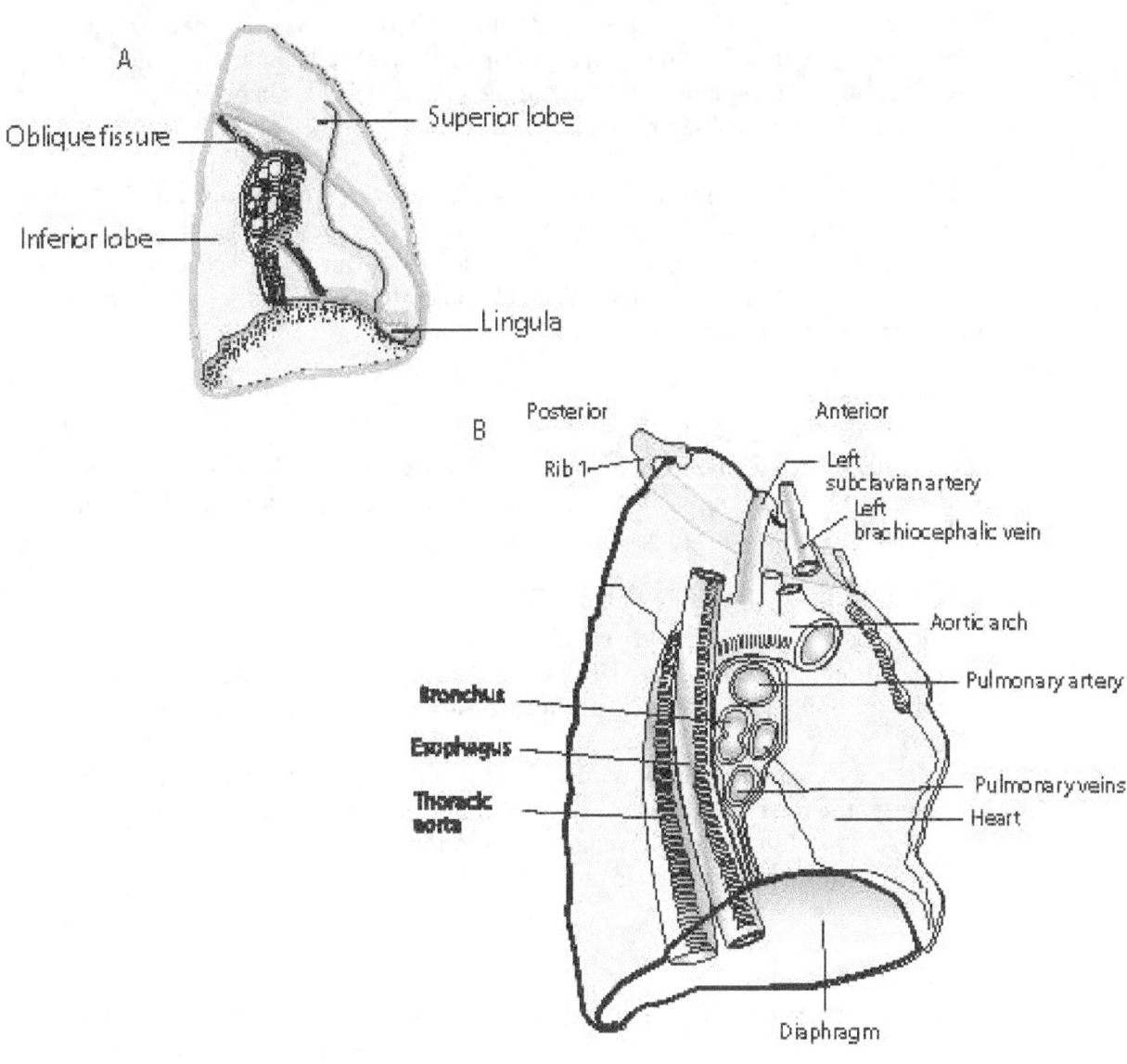

Figure: Structures related to the left lung

Pulmonary ligament
The **mediastinal pleura** surrounding the root of the lung extends downwards beyond the root as a double layered fold called **the pulmonary ligament (pleural sleeve, mesopneumonium or mesentery of the lungs)**. The pulmonary ligament extends from the lower part of the root of the lung as a sickle shaped fold and ends just above the diaphragmatic surface of the lung.

The fold contains a thin layer of loose areolar tissue with a few lymphatics. It **provides a dead space** into which the pulmonary veins can expand during increased venous return as in exercise. The lung roots can also descend into it with the descent of the diaphragm. The pulmonary ligament also serves to retain the lower part of the lung in position

Hilum of the lungs
This is the spot on the medial surface of each lung, at which the structures forming the root (e.g., the main bronchus, pulmonary vessels, bronchial vessels, lymphatic vessels, and nerves) enter and leave the lung. The hilum can be likened to the area of soil where a plant's root enters the ground.

Lobes of the lungs
The right lung is divided into **three lobes** (upper, middle, and lower) by two fissures, the oblique and horizontal fissures. The left lung is divided into **two lobes** by the oblique fissure. The **oblique fissure** cuts the whole thickness of the lung except at the hilum. It passes obliquely crossing the posterior border 6 cm below the apex and the inferior border about 5 cm from the median plane. In the **right lung, the horizontal fissure** passes from the anterior border up to the oblique fissure and separates a wedge shaped middle lobe from the upper lobe. The number of lobes may very in either lung. An accessory lobe, like the *azygos lobe* in the right lung, may also be present.

Borders of the lungs
The anterior margin of the right lung is relatively straight. The anterior border of the left lung has a deep *cardiac notch*. The cardiac notch primarily indents the anteroinferior aspect of the superior lobe of the left lung. The cardiac notch creates a thin tongue like process of the superior lobe, called the *lingula*. The posterior border is thick and ill defined. The inferior border separates the base from the costal and medial surfaces.

Apex, base, and surfaces of the lungs
The **apex** is the blunt superior end of the lung ascending above the level of the 1st costal cartilage into the root of the neck and is covered by the cervical pleura. The **base** is formed by the diaphragmatic surface of the lung and is semilunar and concave. **The diaphragmatic surface of the right lung consists of the middle lobe and the lower lobe. The diaphragmatic surface of the left lung consists of the upper and lower lobe.** The *right lung base* rests on the right dome of the

diaphragm which separates the right lung from the right lobe of the liver. The *left lung base* rests on the left dome of the diaphragm which separates the left lung from the left lobe of the liver, the fundus of the stomach, and the spleen. The costal surface is convex and smooth and is related to the costal pleura. The mediastinal surface is concave. The concavity is more on the left side because $2/3^{rd}$ of the heart is to the left.

Relations of the apex of the lung

Anterior to the apex of the lung is the subclavian artery; **posteriorly**, the cervicothoracic ganglion (stellate ganglion); ventral ramus of the first spinal nerve; and superior intercostal artery. **Laterally**, scalenus medius, and the brachiocephalic trunk, right brachiocephalic vein and trachea are on the right side, while the left subclavian artery and left brachiocephalic vein are on the left. Above the apex of the lung is the cervical pleura and suprapleural membrane.

Differences between the left and right lung

Right lung	Left lung
Two fissures and three lobes	One fissure and two lobes
Anterior border is straight	Anterior border is interrupted by cardiac notch
Larger and heavier and weighs about 700 grams	Smaller and lighter and weighs about 500 grams
Shorter and broader	Longer and narrower

Arterial supply of the lungs

The bronchial vessels

The **bronchial arteries** supply nutrition and oxygen to the bronchial tree and to the lung tissue. Although there is much variation, there are usually two bronchial arteries that run to the left lung, and one to the right lung. The **left bronchial arteries** (superior & inferior) usually arise directly from the thoracic aorta. The **single right bronchial artery** usually arises from one of the following:

- 1) the thoracic aorta at a common trunk with the right 3rd posterior intercostal artery
- 2) the superior bronchial artery on the left side
- 3) any of the upper right intercostal arteries

The bronchial arteries travel with and branch with the bronchi, ending about at the level of the **respiratory bronchioles**. They anastomose with the branches of the pulmonary arteries, and together, they supply the visceral pleura of the lung in the process.

The **bronchial veins** are small vessels that return blood from the larger bronchi and structures at the roots of the lungs. The right side drains into the **azygos vein**, while the left side drains into the **left superior intercostal vein or the accessory hemiazygos vein**.

The bronchial veins are counterparts to the bronchial arteries. The veins, however, do not return all of the blood supplied by the arteries; much of the blood that is carried in the bronchial arteries is returned to the heart via the pulmonary veins.

Note. Bronchial vessels are much smaller than the diameter of the pulmonary vessels.

The pulmonary trunk and its branches

The pulmonary trunk arises from the right ventricle. The pulmonary trunk is anterior and to the left of the ascending aorta. It is about 5cm long and divides into right and left pulmonary arteries just below the arch of the aorta.

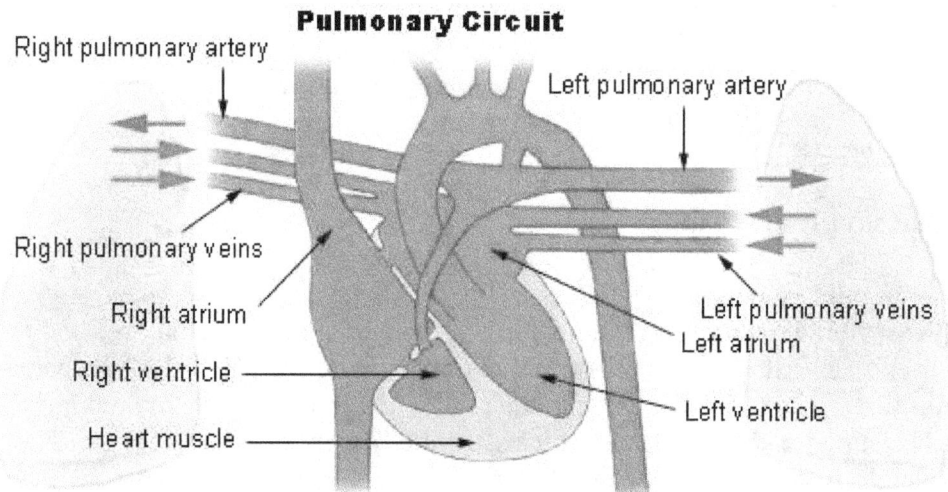

The right pulmonary artery

The right pulmonary artery passes transversely towards the hilum of the right lung, beneath the arch of the aorta; posterior to the ascending aorta and superior vena cava; and anterior to the right principal bronchus.

The left pulmonary artery

The left pulmonary artery is shorter and narrower than the right pulmonary artery; passes in front of the upper part of the descending thoracic aorta and the left principal bronchus. The proximal end of the left pulmonary artery is attached to the arch of the aorta by the ligamentum arteriosum near the bifurcation of the pulmonary trunk. **The ductus arteriosus** becomes the ligamentum arteriosum after birth.

The pulmonary arteries follow the divisions of the bronchi to the level of the terminal bronchiole and forms **pulmonary capillary plexuses**.

Venous drainage of the lungs

The greater part of the venous blood from the lungs is drained by the pulmonary veins.

The venous blood from the first one or two divisions of the bronchi is carried by the bronchial veins. The bronchial veins open into the azygos system of veins.

The pulmonary veins

The **pulmonary veins** carry oxygenated blood from the lungs to the left atrium of the heart. In humans there are four pulmonary veins, two from each lung. They are four in number, two from each lung, and are devoid of valves. They are

- right inferior
- right superior
- left inferior
- left superior
- They commence in a capillary network upon the walls of the air sacs, where they are **continuous with the capillary ramifications of the pulmonary artery**, and, joining together, form one vessel for each alveolus.
- Within the lung, small tributaries of the pulmonary veins run **alone** (i.e., do not run with the bronchial trees, pulmonary arteries, or bronchial arteries).
- Tributaries of the pulmonary veins are found at the periphery of the bronchopulmonary segments (i.e., **intersegmental location).**
- These vessels uniting successively form a single trunk for each lobe, three for the right, and two for the left lung.
- The vein from the middle lobe of the right lung generally unites that from the upper lobe, so that ultimately two trunks from each lung are formed; they perforate the fibrous layer of the pericardium and open separately into the upper and back part of the left atrium.
- Occasionally the three veins on the right side remain separate, and not infrequently the two left pulmonary veins end by a common opening into the left atrium. Therefore, the number of pulmonary veins opening into the left atrium can vary between three and five in the healthy population.
- At the root of the lung, the superior pulmonary vein lies in front of and a little below the pulmonary artery; the inferior is situated at the lowest part of the hilum of the lung and on a plane posterior to the upper vein. Behind the pulmonary artery is the bronchus.
- The right pulmonary veins pass behind the right atrium and superior vena cava; the left in front of the descending thoracic aorta

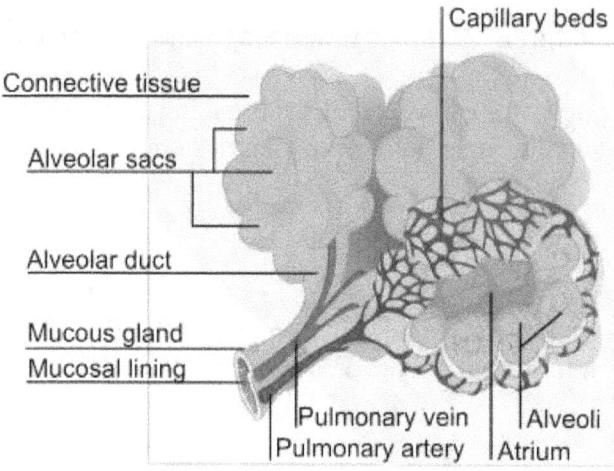

Figure: Microscopic structure of the lung

Notes
- There is anastomosis between the branches of the bronchial artery and the tributaries of the pulmonary veins on the surface of the lung underneath the visceral pleura.
- Tributary of the pulmonary veins passes in the connective tissue septa between the bronchopulmonary segments

Lymphatic drainage of the lungs
The lung has two sets of lymphatic plexuses, the superficial and deep lymphatic plexus. The superficial plexus drains lymph from the visceral pleura and lung parenchyma. The deep lymphatic plexus drains lymph from the bronchi and peribronchial tissue. Both the plexuses drain into the **bronchopulmonary lymph nodes** then to the superior and inferior tracheobronchial lymph nodes. The inferior lobes of both lungs drain to the inferior tracheobronchial (carinal) nodes, which primarily drain to the right side. Most lymph from the lower lobe of the left lung drains to the right side. Lymph from the tracheobronchial lymph nodes passes to the right and left bronchomediastinal lymph trunks. These trunks usually terminate on each side at the venous angles, which are junctions of the subclavian and internal jugular vein.

Nerve supply of the lungs

Parasympathetic	Sympathetic
Derived from the vagus nerve. The fibers are motor to the bronchal muscles. On stimulation causes bronchospasm (decreases the lumen of the bronchus) and increases the secretion of the bronchial glands.	Derived from the lateral (intermediate) horn of the T2-T5 spinal segments. These are inhibitory to the bronchial smooth muscle (causes bronchodilatation) and decrease the secretion of the bronchial glands.

Bronchial tree

78

The trachea divides into left and right principal bronchi. The right principal bronchus is 2.5 cm long. The right principal bronchus is shorter, broader and vertical. The **foreign body** more frequently impacts in the middle and lower lobes because the hyparterial bronchus is in line with the right principal bronchus. The left principal bronchus is 5 cm, narrower and more horizontal than the right principal bronchus hence comparatively less chance of foreign body impaction. Depending on the size and shape of the foreign body, it may be impacted in any part of the respiratory tract from trachea to bronchiole. As an example, a peanut is most likely aspirated into the right lower lobe bronchus of an adult man. It also depends on the age and posture of the individual during aspiration.

Differences between left and right principal bronchi

Left Principal Bronchus	Right Principal Bronchus
Horizontal	Less horizontal
Longer	Shorter
Narrower	Wider
5cm in length	2.5cm in length
Less chance of foreign body impaction	More chance of foreign body impaction

The right principal bronchus has three secondary bronchi: *superior lobar*; *middle lobar*; and *inferior lobar*. The superior lobar bronchus is also called *eparterial bronchus* because this bronchus is superolateral to the right pulmonary artery. The middle lobar bronchus and inferior lobar bronchus together form the *hyparterial bronchus*, which lies inferolateral to the right pulmonary artery.

The left principal bronchus has two secondary bronchi: *superior lobar bronchus*; and *inferior lobar bronchus*. The secondary bronchus divides into *tertiary* or *segmental bronchi*. Each *tertiary bronchus* is destined for a particular *bronchopulmonary segment*.

Bronchopulmonary segments
Bronchopulmonary segments are well-defined sectors of the lung. **Each bronchopulmonary segment contains** a segmental or tertiary bronchus, a branch of the pulmonary artery, and a branch of the bronchial artery, which run together through the central part of the segment. Each of these segments is **pyramidal in shape** with its **apex** directed towards the root of the lung and the bases at the pleural surface. The bronchopulmonary segments are surrounded by a connective tissue septum which is continuous on the surface of the pulmonary pleura. The **intersegmental septum** contains the tributary of the **pulmonary vein and lymphatic vessels.The tributaries of the pulmonary veins form surgical landmarks during segmental resection of the lungs**. The bronchopulmonary segments are independent respiratory segments and the largest subdivision of a lobe.
A bronchopulmonary segment is surgically respectable without disturbing other segments.

Bronchopulmonary segments

Right Lung	Left Lung
Superior lobe 1.Apical, 2.Posterior, 3.Anterior	Superior lobe 1.Apical, 2.Posterior, 3.Anterior, 4.Superior lingular, 5.Inferior lingular
Middle lobe 4. Lateral, 5. Medial	
Inferior lobe 6. Superior, 8.Anterior basal, 7. Medial basal (not seen from lateral view), 9. Lateral basal, 10. Posterior basal	Inferior lobe 6. Superior, 8. Anterior basal, 7. Medial basal (not seen from lateral view), 9. Lateral basal, 10. Posterior basal

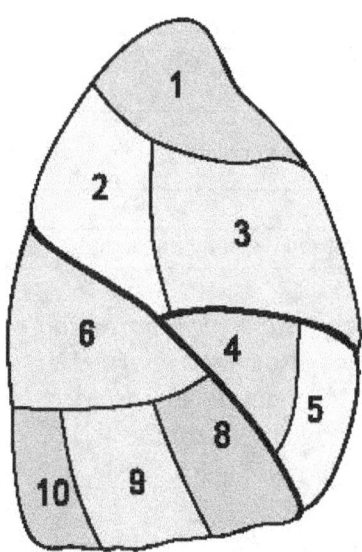

Figure: Right lung bronchopulmonary segments

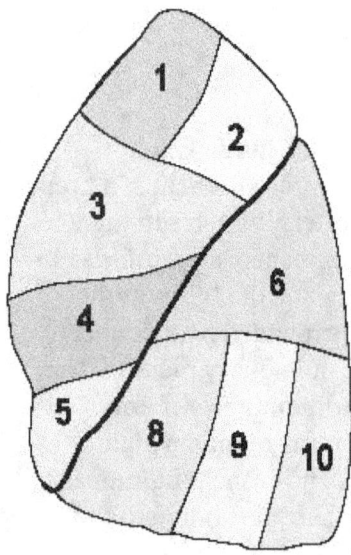

Figure: Left lung bronchopulmonary segments

Notes

In the superior lobe of left lung, the apical and posterior segments typically combined into apicoposterior.

- In the inferior lobe of the left lung, the anterior basal and medial basal bronchopulmonary segments often combined into anteromedial basal.

Auscultation of breath sounds by a stethoscope

1. Breath sounds from the **superior lobes of each lung** can be auscaltated best on the anterosuperior aspect of the thorax.
2. Breath sounds from **inferior lobe** of each lung can be auscaltated best on the posteroinferior aspect of the back.
3. Breath sounds from the **middle lobe of the right lung** can be auscaltated best on the anterior aspect of the thorax lateral to the sternum just **inferior to the right 4th intercostals space.**

Clinical notes

- **Pneumothorax** is the collection of air in the pleural cavity. Pneumothorax is caused by stab wound, rupture of congenital bleb, or iatrogenic (e.g., during endoscopy). In pneumothorax, the mediastinum is shifted towards the opposite side (side away from the side of injury). The affected side gives a dark black shadow in x-ray due to air in the affected side.
- **Pleural effusion** is a collection of fluid in the interpleural space. Pleural effusion is caused by pneumonia, lung cancer, tuberculosis, etc. The affected side gives a white shadow in x-ray due to fluid in the pleural cavity.
- **Pleurisy** is inflammation of the pleura.
  Mesothelioma is a tumor of the pleura. There is a past history of asbestos exposure. Mesothelioma may be benign or malignant. It may happen in the peritoneum of abdomen.
- **Pulmonary embolism (PE)** is a blockage of the pulmonary artery or one of its branches by a substance that has travelled from elsewhere in the body through the bloodstream (embolism). Usually this is due to embolism of a thrombus (blood clot) from the deep veins in the legs. Pulmonary may be blocked by embolus of air, fat or amniotic fluid. The risk of PE is increased in various situations, such as prolonged bed rest, fracture of bones and cancer.
- **Cystic fibrosis** is an inherited disease that causes thick, sticky mucus to build up in the lungs and pancreas. It is one of the most common chronic lung diseases in children and young adults of north European ancestry, and may result in early death. This collection of sticky mucus results in life-threatening lung infections and serious digestion troubles. The disease may also affect the sweat glands and reproductive tracts.
- **Aspiration pneumonia** is common in **alcoholics, postoperative patients** and in **debilitative** patients who lie in the supine position. These groups aspirate vomits or food material very frequently to the superior bronchopulmonary segment of the inferior lobes of the lungs, because these bronchopulmonary segments are most posterior in the supine person.

- **Bronchial asthma** is a common chronic inflammatory disease of the airways characterized by variable and recurring symptoms, reversible airflow obstruction, and bronchospasm. Symptoms include wheezing, coughing, chest tightness, and shortness of breath.

- **Emphysema** is a chronic, progressive obstructive disease of the lungs that primarily causes shortness of breath due to over-inflation and destruction of the alveoli (air sacs in the lung). In people with emphysema, the lung tissue involved in exchange of gases (oxygen and carbon dioxide) is impaired. Emphysema is called an obstructive lung disease because airflow on exhalation is slowed or stopped because over-inflated alveoli do not exchange gases when a person breaths due to little or no movement of gases out of the alveoli.
- **Bronchiectasis** is a disease state defined by localized, irreversible dilation of part of the bronchial tree. It is classified as an **obstructive lung disease**, along with emphysema, bronchitis and cystic fibrosis. Involved bronchi are dilated, inflamed, and easily collapsible, resulting in airflow obstruction and impaired clearance of secretions.
- **Chronic bronchitis** is a chronic inflammation of the bronchi (medium-size airways) in the lungs. It is defined clinically as a persistent cough that produces sputum (phlegm) and mucus, for at least three months in two consecutive years

Histology of the respiratory system

Identifying points of the trachea

- C-shaped incomplete hyaline cartilage rings (16-20). The cartilage is covered adherently by the perichondrium (fibrocellular connective tissue layer over a cartilage).
- The cartilage ring is completed posteriorly by smooth muscle called trachealis.
- The luminal surface of the trachea is lined by pseudostratified ciliated columnar epithelium.
- The mucosa (epithelium and lamina propria) also contains basal, goblet (unicellular mucus gland), ciliated, brush, and **DNES** cells (Diffuse Neuro Endocrine System).
- The submucosa is rich in seromucus glands particularly where the cartilage is deficient.
- The C-shaped cartilages are connected to each other by dense connective tissue (anular ligament).

Identifying points of secondary (intrapulmonary) bronchi
- Plates of hyaline cartilage (bronchi of all sizes contain some cartilage)
- Helically-oriented smooth muscle
- Lined by pseudostratified ciliated columnar epithelium with basal cells, goblet cells, brush cells and DNES cells
- Seromucus glands

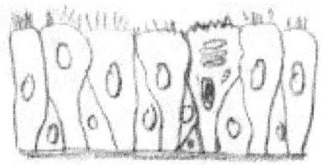

Pseudostratifed ciliated columnar epithelium

Bronchiole

Bronchioles are also known as bronchiole-terminal bronchiole-respiratory bronchiole and are distal airways located between the cartilages walled bronchi and the site where the ciliated epithelium ceases.

- Bronchiole has no cartilage and no glands (occasionally large bronchiole has goblet cells)
- Bronchiole has smooth muscle
- The lining epithelium of the bronchioles changes gradually from simple columnar→simple cuboidal→simple squamous (bronchiole→terminal bronchiole→respiratory bronchiole)
- The number of ciliated cells also decreases gradually
- Bronchioles contain clara cells

Clara cells

Clara cells are non-ciliated columnar cells with dome shaped apices. They are most numerous in the terminal bronchiole. They have secretory granules and secrete proteins that **protect** the bronchiolar lining against oxidative pollutants and inflammation. Clara cells undergo mitosis to replace the bronchiolar epithelium.

Alveoli of the lung

Alveoli are terminal units within the lung used for gas exchange. They are **lined** by highly attenuated **simple squamous epithelium**. Type I is simple squamous and Type II pneumocyte is cuboidal cells. There are no glands in the alveoli. They are supported by Type III collagen and elastic fibers, having a diameter of 200μm and alveolar macrophages.

Immotile Cilia Syndrome (Kartageners Syndrome)

Kartageners Syndrome is a disorder that causes **infertility** and chronic respiratory tract infection (e.g., sinusitis, bronchitis, and emphysema) in both sexes. The syndrome is caused by immobility of the cilia and flagella, induced in some cases by deficiency of **dynein**, a protein normally present in the cilia, which participates in the ciliary movement. Immotile cilia syndrome may be associated with **dextrocardia**.

Surfactant

Surfactant is secreted from the **pneumocyte type II cells** within the alveoli. Pneumocyte Type II cells are cuboidal or rounded cells rich in mitochondria and endoplasmic reticulum. Surfactant is a mixture of phospholipids. Surfactant decreases the surface tension of the alveoli. Absence of surfactant causes alveolar collapse and *respiratory distress syndrome* of children, primary a condition in premature infants.

Pancoast tumor of the lung

Tumor at the apex of the lung is called *pancoast tumor (a non-small cell lung cancer)*. The pancoast tumor may compress several structures at the root of the neck and may cause a number of clinical scenarios as follows.

1. Sympathetic truck compression---results in **Horner's syndrome**.
2. Recurrent laryngeal nerve compression---results in **hoarseness of voice**
3. Phrenic nerve compression---results in paralysis of a dome of the diaphragm (**hemidiaphragm**)
4. Subclavian artery compression---results in **diminished pulse** in the extremity
5. Brachiocephalic or subclavian vein compression---results in **venous engorgement** and edema of the face and arm on one side
6. Thoracic duct compression is possible in left sided pancoast tumor---results in **edema** below

Horner's syndrome

Horner's syndrome is a clinical syndrome characterized by: **ptosis** (drooping of the upper eyelid due to paralysis of the superior tarsal muscle); **miosis** (pupillary constriction); **anhydrosis** (lack of sweating in the affected side of the forehead); **enopthalmos** (relative sinking of the eyeball in the orbit); redness; and increased temperature of the skin (vasodilation). Horner's syndrome results from interruption of a cervical sympathetic trunk and is manifested by the lack of sympathetically stimulated functions on the ipsilateral side of the head. Horner's syndrome is caused by **apical tumor** of the lung (Pancoast tumor); and **injury to the carotid arteries** (because sympathetic nerves passes over the carotid arteries). On rare occasion, it may be congenital.

EMBRYOLOGY OF THE RESPIRATORY SYSTEM

The lungs **begin** to develop in the **fourth** intrauterine week and **complete maturation** by 8 to 10 years after birth. The respiratory system originates as a ventral foregut diverticulum that undergoes a controlled series of branching. The epithelium of the larynx, trachea, bronchi, and alveoli originates in the **endoderm**. The cartilages, muscles, and connective tissue components develops from the **splanchnopleuric mesoderm**.

Tracheoesophageal septum separates the trachea from the foregut, dividing the foregut into lung bud anteriorly and the esophagus posteriorly. The larynx maintains communication between the foregut and the lung bud. The lung bud develops into two principal bronchi. The right principal bronchi forms three secondary bronchi and three lobes; the left principal bronchi forms two secondary bronchi and two lobes. **Faulty partitioning** of the foregut by the esophagotracheal septum causes **esophageal atresia and tracheoesophageal fistula**.

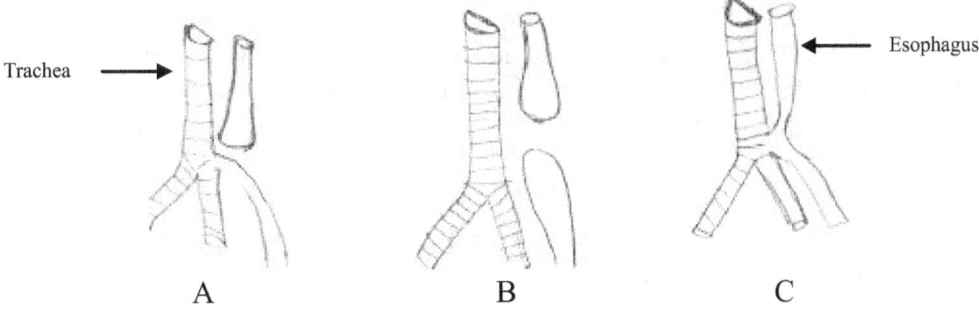

Trachea →

← Esophagus

A   B   C

Tracheoesophageal fistula

Maturation of the lungs during intrauterine life
Maturation of the lungs during intrauterine period is divided into **four periods**: **Pseudoglandular** period (5-16 weeks) - cells are tall columnar; **Canalicular period** (16-26 weeks) - cells are low columnar; **Terminal sac** period (26 weeks to birth) - cells become cuboidal to flattened; and **Alveolar period** (32 weeks to 8 years) - cells are simple squamous.

In the **terminal sac period**, the flat cells (type I alveolar epithelial cells) associate intimately with blood and lymph capillaries. By the end of the 6th month, approximately **17th generations** of subdivision have formed.

During postnatal life, six additional divisions form before the bronchial tree reaches its final shape. In the 7th month, gas exchange between the blood and air in the primitive alveoli is possible. The secondary bronchi divide repeatedly in a **dichotomous fashion**, forming ten tertiary (segmental) bronchi in the right lung and 8 in the left lung, creating the bronchopulmonary segment of the adult lung. Hence, the **number of alveoli** in a newborn is less than an adolescent. The **respiratory problems** (e.g., bronchial asthma) in an infant or toddler might disappear at puberty, and may be due to an increase in the number of alveoli.

Before birth the lungs are filled with fluid with little protein, some mucus, and surfactant, which is produced by **type II alveolar epithelial cells** (also called pneumocyte type II cell). Surfactant forms a phospholipids coat on the alveolar epithelium. **Surfactant** prevents the collapse of the alveoli during expiration by decreasing the surface tension. Absence of surfactant in the premature baby causes Respiratory Distress Syndrome due to collapse of the alveoli (hyaline membrane disease).

Growth of the lungs after birth

There is increase in the number of the bronchiole and alveoli. There is no increase in the size of the alveoli. New alveoli are formed during first 10 years of postnatal life.

Congenital anomalies

Congenital cyst in the lung may be singular or numerous. There may be **associated** polycystic **kidney disease and berry aneurysm of the 'Circle of Willis'.**
 Tracheoesophageal fistula is associated with **faulty partitioning by tracheoesophageal septum**. There are different types of tracheoesophageal fistula depending on the location of the esophageal atresia and communication to the trachea.

"VACTERL" is the association of a number of congenital anomalies.
    V - vertebral anomalies
    A - anal atresia
    T - tracheoesophageal fistula
    E - esophageal atresia
    R - renal anomalies.
    L - limb defects

Objective Questions (Set-15)

1. What is meant by principal, secondary and tertiary bronchus?
2. To which lobes of the lung do the eparterial and hyparterial bronchus go?
3. Describe horizontal and transverse fissures of the lungs.
4. What is the lingula? In which bronchopulmonary segment is it present?
5. Which artery provides oxygenated blood to the bronchi and pulmonary connective tissue?
6. What is the nerve supply of the lung?
7. What are the effects of sympathetic and parasympathetic innervations to the lung?
8. What is the blood supply of the lung?
9. What is pneumothorax?
10. Is it possible to have pneumothorax due to stab wound at the root of the neck 2.5 cm medial to the sternal end of the clavicle?
11. In what direction does the mediastinum shift in pneumothorax?
12. What is Kartagener's syndrome?
13. What is Horner's syndrome?
14. What is situs inversus?
15. Name the structures which are related to the apex of the lung.
16. What are the contents of the root of the lung and how are they arranged?
17. Which nerve passes anterior to the root of the lung?
18. Which nerve passes behind the root of the lung?
19. What is pulmonary ligament and what is its function?
20. What is the lymphatic drainage of the lung?
21. What are the impressions on the mediastinal surfaces of the right lung and left lung?

Multiple Choice Questions (Set-15)

1. Select an INCORRECT statement
   A. The epithelium of the trachea, bronchi and alveoli are endodermal in origin.
   B. The esophagus and trachea are separated by ingrowth of the esophagotracheal ridge.
   C. The respiratory diverticulum from the foregut forms the lung bud.
   D. The parietal pleura develops from the splanchnic mesoderm.

2. The horizontal fissure of the right lung extends from the oblique fissure along _____ anteriorly.
   A. right 2nd rib and costal cartilage
   B. right 4th rib and costal cartilage

C. right 6th rib and costal cartilage
D. right 7th rib and costal cartilage

3. Vagus nerve stimulation causes which of the following to the lungs?
   A. Bronchoconstriction
   B. Bronchodilation
   C. Vasoconstriction
   D. Decreased secretion from the bronchial glands

4. A bronchopulmonary segment of the lung contains_____.
   A. trachea
   B. principal bronchus
   C. secondary bronchus
   D. tertiary bronchus

5. An INCORRECT statement about the horizontal fissure is that the horizontal fissure
   A. begins at the level of 4th costal cartilage
   B. passes horizontally
   C. meets the oblique fissure at the midaxillary line
   D. is present in both the left and right lung

6. Which of the following bronchopulmonary segments are mostly involved in aspiration pneumonia?
   A. Apical bronchopulmonary segment of upper lobes of left and right lung
   B. Lateral bronchopulmonary segment of the middle lobe of the right lung
   C. Medial bronchopulmonary segment of the middle lobe of the right lung
   D. Superior bronchopulmonary segment of the lower lobes of the left and right lung

7. Select an INCORRECT statement about the blood supply of the lung.
   A. Venous blood from the terminal bronchioles is drained by the bronchial veins.
   B. The tributaries of the pulmonary artery pass between the bronchopulmonary segments.
   C. The two left bronchial arteries are branches of the descending thoracic aorta.
   D. The bronchial arteries provide nutrition to the bronchi and pulmonary tissue.

8. Situs inversus, bronchiectasis, and abnormal spermatozoa are associated with which of the following syndrome?
   A. Horner's syndrome
   B. Fragile X syndrome
   C. Klinefelters syndrome
   D. Kartagener syndrome
   E. Down syndrome

9. Drooping of the eyelid seen in Horner's syndrome is caused by paralysis of_____muscle
   A. orbicularis oculi
   B. fronto-occipitalis
   C. levator palpabrae superioris
   D. superior tarsal

10. Which of the following structures is related to the posterior aspect of the apex of the lung?
   A. Subclavian artery
   B. Brachicephalic trunk
   C. Trachea
   D. Scalenus medius
   E. Stellate ganglion

11. What is the lining epithelium of the luminal surface of the trachea?
   A. Pseudostratified ciliated columnar
   B. Stratified squamous
   C. Transitional
   D. Simple squamous
   E. Simple cuboidal

12. What is the lining epithelium of the alveoli of the lung?
   A. Stratified columnar
   B. Simple cuboidal
   C. Simple squamous
   D. Transitional
   E. Stratified squamous

13. Hyaline membrane disease is caused by lack of secretion of surfactant from which of the following cells?
   A. Pneumocyte type I cells
   B. Pneumocyte type II cells
   C. Goblet cells
   D. DNES cells
   E. Alveolar macrophages

14. Lingula is located in the_____.
   A. upper lobe of the left lung
   B. middle lobe of the right lung
   C. lower lobe of the left lung
   D. upper lobe of the right lung

MCQ (Set-15) Answers: 1. D; 2. B; 3. A; 4. D; 5. D; 6. D; 7. A; 8. D; 9. D; 10. E; 11. A; 12. C; 13. B; 14. A

The Heart

The *heart* is a hollow muscular organ situated in the ***middle mediastinum.*** The heart has four chambers: the right atrium; the left atrium; the right ventricle; and the left ventricle. The atria are **receiving chambers** and the ventricles are **discharging chambers**. The heart is enclosed within the pericardium. Circulation of the blood occurs through the heart and lungs.

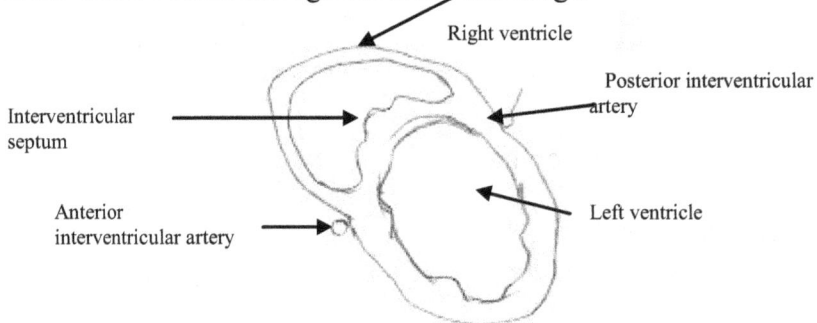

Transverse section of the heart ventricles

Right atrium

The *right atrium* receives deoxygenated blood from the body through the superior vena cava, inferior vena cava, and coronary sinus. The right ventricle receives deoxygenated blood from the right atrium and pumps the blood to the lungs for oxygenation through the pulmonary trunk.

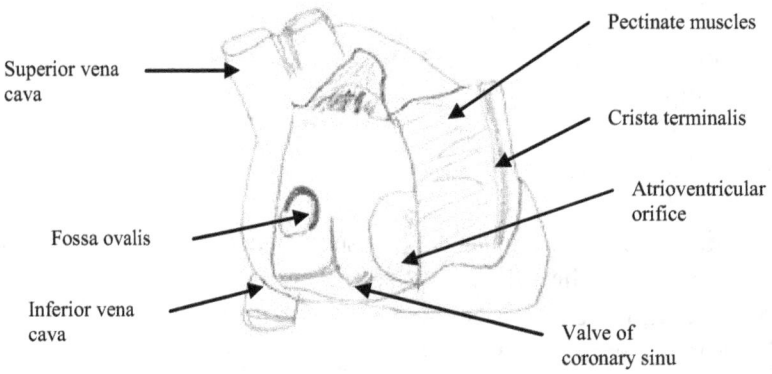

Interior of right atrium

Left atrium

The *left atrium* receives oxygenated blood from the lungs through the pulmonary veins. The left ventricle receives blood from the left atrium. The oxygenated blood of the left ventricle is distributed to the body through the aorta.

Surface anatomy of the heart

Right border can be illustrated by drawing a line with a slight convexity toward the right connecting the right second costal cartilage (1 cm from the right lateral sternal border) and the right 6th costal cartilage (1 cm from the right lateral sternal border).

Inferior border can be illustrated by drawing a line connecting the right 6th costal cartilage (1 cm from the right sternal border) and the left 5th intercostal space on the left side of the midclavicular line.

Left border can be illustrated by drawing a line connecting the left 5th intercostal space on the left side of the midclavicular line and the left 2nd costal cartilage along the left sternal border.

Superior border can be illustrated by drawing a line connecting the inferior margin of the 2nd costal cartilage along the left sternal border and inferior margin of the 2nd costal cartilage along the the right sternal border.

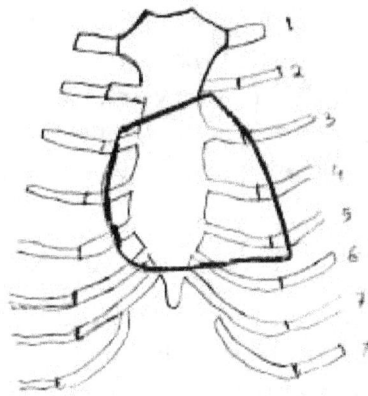

Surface Anatomy of the Heart

The surfaces of the heart
The heart has **four surfaces**: sternocostal; diaphragmatic; right pulmonary; and left pulmonary. The anterior or **sternocostal surface** is formed mainly by the right ventricle. The **inferior or diaphragmatic surface** is formed mainly by the left ventricle and partly by the right ventricle. The diaphragmatic surface is related to the **central tendon** of **the diaphragm**. The **right pulmonary surface** is formed mainly by the right atrium. The **left pulmonary surface** is formed mainly by the left ventricle and left auricle.

Borders (Margins) of the heart
Right and left pulmonary surfaces represent the *right and left margins* of the heart. The *inferior margin* is a sharp edge between the anterior surface and the diaphragmatic surface. The inferior margin is formed by the right ventricle mostly and by the left ventricle near the apex of the heart. The *obtuse margin* separates the anterior and left pulmonary surfaces. The *superior border* is formed by the left and right atria and auricles. Posterior to the aorta and pulmonary trunk and anterior to the superior vena cava, this border forms the inferior boundary of the transverse pericardial sinus.

Precordium is the anterior chest wall which covers sternocostal surface of the heart.

Area of superficial cardiac dullness

Percussion of the anterior chest wall reveals a variable area of dullness from 4th to 6th costal cartilage that extends approximately 3.5 cm from the left border to the sternum. This area lies between the left sternal border and the cardiac notch of the left lung along its anterior border. It is roughly triangular in shape and corresponds to the part of the sternocostal surface of the heart covered by the pericardium and double layer of pleura that is close to the anterior chest wall and not covered by left lung

Coronary sulcus (atrioventricular groove)

Externally the atria are demarcated from the ventricles by the coronary or atrioventricular groove also called *coronary sulcus*. The **coronary sulcus contains main trunks of the coronary arteries,** coronary sinus, and circumflex branch of the left coronary artery. The right and left ventricles are demarcated from each other by anterior and posterior **interventricular grooves.**

Structure of the wall of the heart

The walls of each heart chamber consist of three layers: the *endocardium*; **the** *myocardium*; and the *epicardium*. The **endocardium** is a thin internal layer made up of endothelium and subendothelial connective tissue which lines the membrane of the heart and also covers its valves. The *myocardium* is a thick helical middle layer composed of cardiac muscle characterized by cylindrical pattern with one or two centrally located nuclei and junctional complex (intercalated disc). The *epicardium* is a thin external layer (mesothelium) formed by the visceral layer of serous pericardium. The lining epithelium of the endocardium and epicardium is simple squamous

Valves of the heart

The valves of the heart have cusps. Each cusp has inner fibrous tissue lined by endothelium on both surfaces. The *right atrioventricular, aortic,* and *pulmonary* valves have **three cusps.** The *left atrioventricular* valve has **two cusps.** The left atrioventricular valve is called *mitral valve* (**like the miter of a bishop**). The right atrioventricular valve is called *tricuspid valve*. Both the aortic and pulmonary valves are called *semilunar valves*. The pulmonary valve is anterior to the aortic valve. The **mitral valve** is the valve **mostly affected rheumatic heart disease.**

Anatomical locations of the valves of the heart

The *pulmonary valve* is located posterior to the **left 3rd sternochondral junction.** The *aortic valve* is posterior to the midsternal line at the level of the **3rd intercostal space.** The *tricuspid valve* is located posterior to the midsternal line at the level of the **5th sternocostal junction.** The *mitral valve* is located posterior to the left **4th sternochondral junction.**

Sites for auscultation of each of the cardiac valves

The **aortic valve area** is at the right 2nd intercostal space along the sternal border. The **pulmonary valve area** is at the left 2nd intercostal space along the sternal border. The **tricuspid valve area** is at the left 5th intercostal space along the

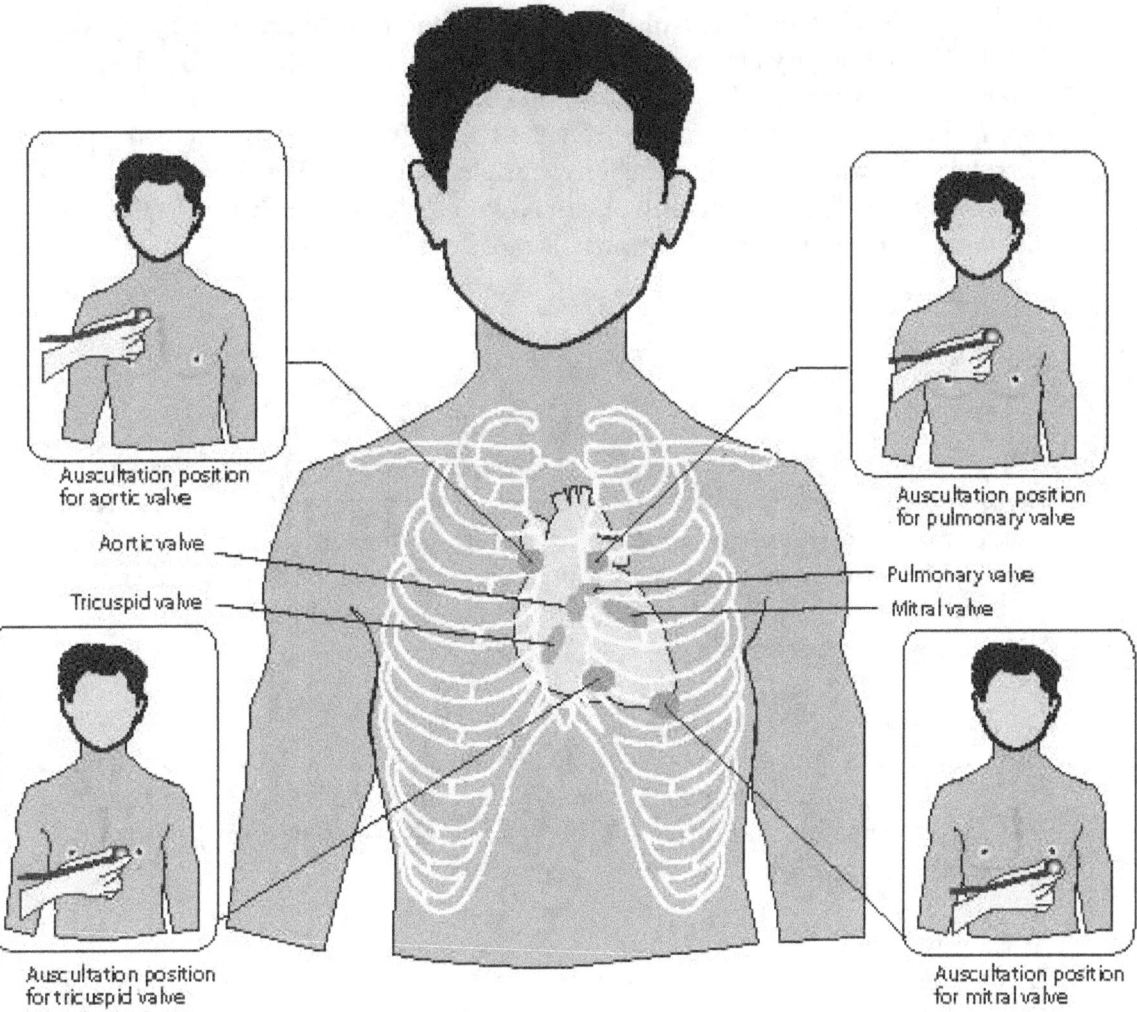

sternal border. The **mitral valve area** is located at the left 5th intercostal space to the left side of the midclavicular line.

Figure: Location of the heart valves, and auscaltation

Valve projection areas

The heart sound is the loudest or most clearly heard by a stethoscope over the specific valve projection areas. The **aortic area** is where the **second heart sound (S2)** can be best heard. **Tricuspid area** is where the **first heart sound (S1)** is found. The pulmonary area is where the second heart sound (S2) is found. The **mitral area** is where the **first heart sound (S1)** is best heard. *Apex beat (apical impulse)* is the impulse that results from the apex of the heart being forced against the anterior thoracic wall when the left ventricle contracts. **The apex beat transmits the closure of the mitral valve.** *Point of maximal impulse (PMI) is the point at which the apical impulse is most readily seen or felt.*

Heart sounds

The *first heart sound* is caused by the closure of the mitral and tricuspid valves. The *second heart sound* is caused by the closure of the aortic and pulmonary valves. The *third heart sound* is the initial part of the ventricular diastole and atrial contraction. The *fourth heart sound* is the last part of the ventricular diastole and atrial contraction.

Cardiac cycle

The synchronous pumping actions of the two atrioventricular (AV) pumps (right and left chambers) constitute the *cardiac cycle*. The cycle begins with a period of ventricular elongation and filling (*diastole*) and ends with a period of shortening and emptying (*systole*).

Apex of the heart

The *apex of the heart* is formed by the inferolateral part of the left ventricle. The apex of the heart lies posterior to the left 5th intercostal space in adults, approximately 9 cm (a hand's breadth from the median plane). The apex remains motionless throughout the cardiac cycle. The sound of the mitral valve closure is maximal in the apex, hence is referred to as the *apex beat*. The **apex beat** is the impulse that results from the apex of the heart being forced against the anterior chest wall when the left ventricle contracts. The apex beat may be auscultated through the thoracic wall over the apex of the heart. The location of the apex beat varies in position from person to person. It may be located in the 4th or 5th intercostal spaces, approximately 6 - 10 cm from the midsternal line.

Dextrocardia is a condition where the heart is located on the opposite side of the thorax. In dextrocardia, the apex of the heart is located in the right 5th intercostal space, approximately 9 cm from the median plane. Dextrocardia may be **isolated** or may be **linked** with **situs inversus**, where other internal organs are transposed. Isolated dextrocardia is usually complicated by severe cardiac anomalies, such as single ventricle and arterial transposition.

Base of the heart

The base of the heart is located at the posterosuperior aspect of the heart. This is directly opposite the apex. It is **formed mainly by the left atrium with contribution from the right atrium.** It lies anterior to the bodies of T6-T9 vertebrae separated by the esophagus, aorta, pericardium and the oblique pericardial sinus. The base of the heart extends from the bifurcation of the pulmonary trunk to the coronary sinus.

Development of the right atrium

The heart is formed from the fusion of two **endothelial heart tubes** and develops from the **splanchnopleuric mesoderm**. The right atrium has two parts: rough and smooth. The **rough part** forms from the primitive atrium as represented by the right auricle and pectinate muscles. The **smooth part** develops from the absorption of the sinus venosus as represented by the sinus venarum. There are three structures that open into the sinus venarum: superior vena cava; inferior vena cava; and coronary sinus. The remnants of the sinus venosus are represented by the sinus venosus, coronary sinus, and oblique vein of left atrium.

Right atrium of the heart

The right atrium is the right upper chamber of the heart. It drains blood to the right ventricle through the *tricuspid valve*. The right atrium forms the right border of the heart and part of the superior border, sternocostal surface and base of the heart. The **right atrium receives** venous blood through the superior vena, inferior vena cava, and coronary sinus. A vertical ridge, the *crista terminalis or terminal crest*, separates the rough part from the smooth part of the interior surface of the right atrium. The opening of the coronary sinus, a short venous trunk receiving most of the cardiac veins, is between the vestibule of the right atrioventricular orifice, oval fossa, and the inferior vena cava orifice. The **coronary sinus** is often guarded by a thin semicircular valve called *Thebesius' valve*. The superior vena cava has **no valves**. The inferior vena cava has a rudimentary valve called the *Eustachian valve*, which is a semilunar crescent of tissue. It has no function after birth. It is variable in size, and is occasionally absent. The interatrial septum separating the atria has an oval thumbprint-size depression called the *oval fossa or fossa ovalis*. It is a vestige of the *oval foramen* or *foramen ovale* valve in the fetus. The floor of the oval fossa is formed by the *septum primum*, the primary atrial septum. The rim of the fossa ovalis is called *limbus of fossa ovalis* and is formed from the *septum secundum*. The upper part of the fossa ovalis may have a small slit in 30% of normal hearts called *pin-probe patency*. This is a harmless heart anomaly.

Triangle of Koch

The *Triangle of Koch* is located in the right atrium. It is bounded by the *tendon of Todaro*, the *ostium of the coronary sinus* and the *septal cusp* of the tricuspid valve. The tendon of Todaro is a tendinous structure that runs into the septum between the coronary sinus and fossa ovalis from junction between the valves of the inferior vena cava and coronary sinus.Traiangle of Koch contains **A-V node** beneath its floor.

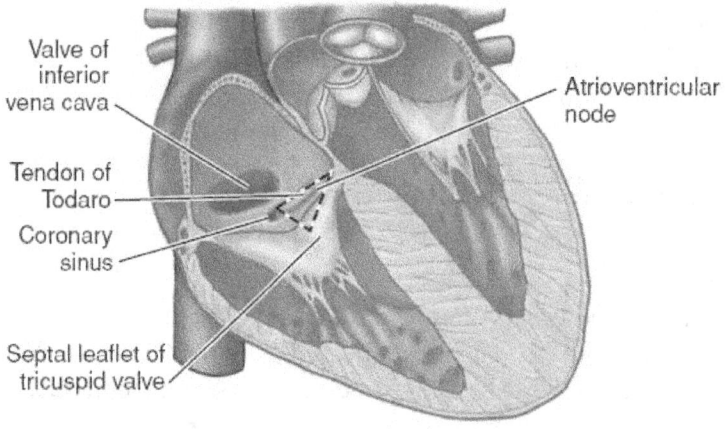

Figure: Triangle of Koch in the right atrium

Left atrium of the heart
The base of the heart is mainly formed by the left atrium. The left atrium makes up the left posterosuperior part of the heart. It receives oxygenated blood through four pulmonary veins. These four pulmonary veins are absorbed in the left atrium during intrauterine life and form the **smooth walled** part of the left atrium. The blood from the left atrium reaches the left ventricle by the mitral (left atrioventricular) valve. The left atrioventricular valve is a bicuspid valve called *mitral valve* because it looks like the mitre of a Bishop. The left atrium has a **rough part** in the left auricle and in the vestibule of the mitral valve. The left auricle is an earlike process and contains pectinate muscle. The wall of the left atrium is slightly thicker than the right atrium. The rough part develops from the **primitive atrium** and contains pectinate muscle like the right atrium. A crescent shaped ridge is seen in the interatrial septum along the interior of the left atrium represent the valve of the foramen ovale, called *falx septi*. The ridge outlines the *fossa lunata* corresponding to the fossa ovalis.

Endocrine functions of the heart
Heart muscles, in particular the right atrial muscle contains granules containing atrial natriuretic peptides **(ANP)** also called atrial natriuretic factor **(ANF),** a hormone that lowers blood pressure. This hormone act by decreasing reabsorption of sodium and water from the renal tubules.

Right ventricle
The right ventricle forms most of the anterior surface of the heart and a portion of the diaphragmatic surface. The outflow part of the right ventricle, which leads to the pulmonary trunk, is the *conus arteriosus* or *infundibulum.* This area has smooth walls and develops from the embryonic *bulbus cordis*. The inflow portion of the right ventricle has numerous irregular muscular structures called *trabeculae carnae*. A few trabeculae carnae (papillary muscles) have only one end attached to the ventricular surface, while the other end serves as the point of attachment for tendon-like fibrous cord, the *chordae tendinae*. The chordae tendinae connect the free edges of the cusps of the tricuspid valve to the papillary muscles.

Left ventricle

The left ventricle forms the apex of the heart and nearly all of its left surface and border, and most of the diaphragmatic surface. The wall of the left ventricle is **three times as thick** as that of the right ventricle. The trabeculae carnae of the left ventricle is finer and more numerous than that of the right ventricle. The cavity of the left ventricle is conical.

The anterior and posterior papillary muscles are **larger** than that of the right ventricle.

Papillary muscles of the right ventricle

There are **three papillary muscles** in the right ventricle corresponding to the cusp of the tricuspid valve, the anterior, posterior, and septal papillary muscles. The *anterior papillary muscle* arises from the anterior wall of the right ventricle. Its tendinous cords attach to the anterior and posterior cusps of the tricuspid valve. The *posterior papillary muscle* arises from the inferior wall of the right ventricle. Its tendinous cords attach to the posterior and septal cusp of the tricuspid valve. The *septal papillary muscle* arises from the interventricular septum. This tendinous cord attach to the anterior and septal cusps of the tricuspid valve. The papillary muscles function to prevent the valve cusp from entering the atrium during systole.

Septomarginal Trabecula/Moderator Band

The *septomarginal trabeculae or moderator band* is a curved muscular bundle that traverses the right ventricular chamber from the inferior part of the interventricular septum to the base of the anterior papillary muscle. The moderator band **carries** part of the right branch of the **atrioventricular bundle**, a part of the conducting system of the heart to the anterior papillary muscle. This **shortcut** seems to facilitate conduction time, allowing coordinated contraction of the anterior papillary muscle.

Supraventricular Crest

The *supraventricular crest* is a thick muscular ridge present in the right ventricle. It separates the rough muscular wall of the inflow part of the right ventricle from the smooth walled conus arteriosus, the outflow part of the right ventricle.

Interventricular Septum

The *interventricular septum*, composed of **membranous and muscular parts**, is an obliquely placed partition between the right and left ventricles. The upper part of the interventricular septum is membranous and is the common site of ventricular septal defect (**VSD**). VSD may be an isolated defect or it may be a component of the *Fallots Tetralogy*. The interventricular septum is supplied by anterior interventricular artery and posterior interventricular artery.

Conducting system of the heart

The conducting system of the heart is made up of **specialized cardiac muscles** (myocardium) that produce impulses. The components of the conducting system are as follows.

- Sinoatrial (S-A node)
- Atrioventricular node (A-V node)
- Bundle of His
- Left and Right Bundles
- Purkinje Fibers.

Component of the conducting system of the heart	Location
S-A node	The **sinoatrial** node (pacemaker) is located at the junction of the superior vena cava and the right atrium at the upper end of the crista terminalis
A-V node	The **AV node** is located beneath the endocardium of the medial wall of the right atrium just in front of the opening of the coronary sinus and immediately above the tricuspid valve ring(triangle of Koch)
Bundle of His	**The bundle of His** is located on the upper end of the interventricular septum
Right and left branch of bundle	They are located on each side of the interventricular septum
Purkinje fibers	In the wall of the left and right ventricles

Sinoatrial node

The sinoatrial node is referred to as the *pacemaker* of the heart. The blood supply of the conducting system of the heart is the left and right coronary arteries. An *Artificial Cardiac Pacemaker* is required when the S-A node becomes defective. An artificial pacemaker is approximately the size of a pocket watch and is implanted subcutaneously in the chest wall. It consists of a pulse generator, a wire (lead), and an electrode. The **electrode** is passed through a vein to the SVC, right atrium, then to the **trabeculae carneae of the right ventricle**. A person can survive for many years with an artificial pacemaker.

Cardiac arrhythmias

Cardiac arrhythmias are a variation of the normal rhythm of heart beat. They result from defect or damage to the conducting system of the heart.

Cardiac skeleton

The *cardiac skeleton* is composed of dense connective tissue having three components: **annuli fibrosi; trigonum fibrosum; and septum membranaceum**. The annuli fibrosi is connective tissue formed around the base of the aorta, pulmonary trunk, and the atrioventricular orifices. The trigonum fibrosum is present around the aortic valve. The septum membranaceum forms the upper portion of the interventricular septum. The cardiac skeleton **serves four major functions.** The first is the attachment of the valves. The second is the attachment of cardiac muscles. The third is discontinuity between the myocardium of the atria and ventricle, thus ensuring a rhythmic and cyclic beating of the heart, controlled by the conduction mechanism of the atrioventricular bundles. The fourth is to provide a structural framework for the heart. The cardiac skeleton is **perforated** by atrioventricular bundle.

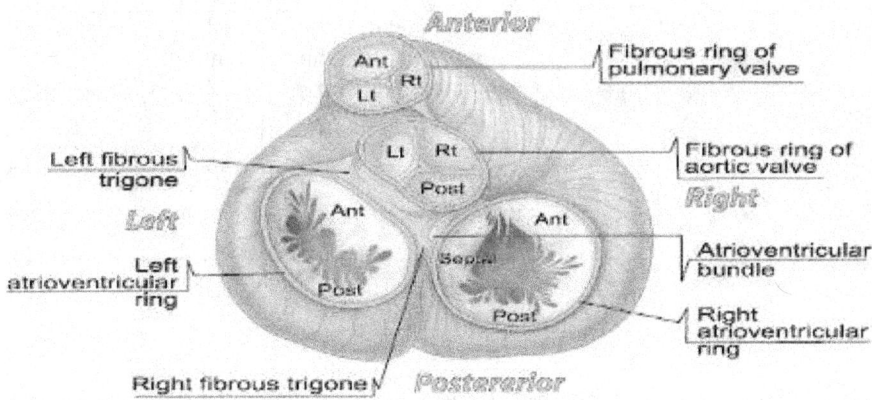

Figure: Skeleton of the heart

Arterial blood supply of the heart
The heart is supplied by the left and right coronary arteries. The left coronary artery arises from the left aortic sinus of the ascending aorta. The right coronary artery arises from the right aortic sinus of the ascending aorta. The coronary arteries are functional end arteries. There is anastomosis between the branches of the coronary arteries, but they are not sufficient enough to prevent myocardial infarction. There are variations in the distribution of the coronary arteries.

Major arterial supply of the heart

Artery	Origin	Course	Distribution
Left coronary artery	Arises from left aortic sinus of the ascending aorta	Runs forward and to the left, emerges between the pulmonary trunk and left auricle, gives two major branches: 1. Anterior interventricular artery 2. Circumflex artery	1. Left Atrium 2. Left and Right ventricles 3. Interventricular septum 4. AV bundle *Left coronary artery is larger than right coronary artery
Right coronary artery	Arises from right aortic sinus of the ascending aorta	Passes forward and to the right to emerge between the root of the pulmonary trunk and the right auricle, gives two major branches--- 1. Right marginal artery 2. Posterior interventricular artery	1. Right atrium 2. Right and left ventricles 3. SA node 4. AV node and most of the conducting system of the heart
Anretior intervantricular artery also called left anterior descending artery (LAD)	Left coronary artery	Passes along the anterior interventricular groove	Right and left ventricles and the anterior two third of the interventricular septum

99

Posterior interventricular artery	Right coronary artery	Passes along the posterior interventricular groove	Right and left ventricles and the and the posterior one third of the interventricular septum
Circumflex branch	Left coronary artery	Winds round the left border of the heart and continues in the left posterior coronary sinus	Left atrium and left ventricle
Right marginal artery	Right coronary artery	Passes along the inferior margin of the heart	Right ventricle

Notes

- The **three most common** sites of coronary artery occlusion in **myocardial infarction (MI)** are the *anterior interventricular branch* (LAD) of the *left coronary artery* (in 40-50% cases), the *right coronary artery* (in 30-40% cases), and the *circumflex branch of the left coronary artery* (in 15-20% cases).

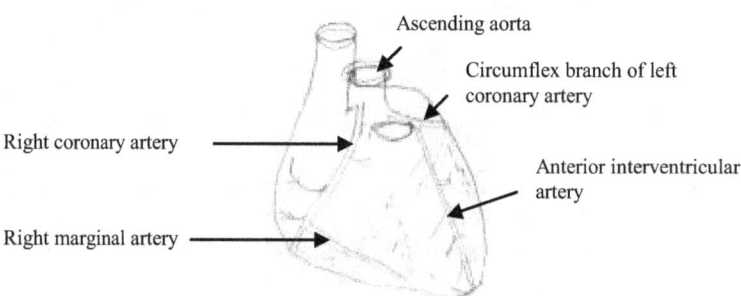

Principal arteries of the heart

Myocardial infarction

Myocardial infarction (MI) is an acute condition resulting from **sudden occlusion** of coronary circulation due to release of the atheromatous debris. In MI there is **necrosis** (nuclear death of the cells) of the myocardium and arrhythmia, due to lack of blood supply to the conducting system of the heart. In slow occlusion of the coronary arteries (e.g.,atherosclerosis) there is establishment of collateral anastomotic channels from the right and left coronary arteries, vasa vasorum of the aorta, pulmonary arteries, internal thoracic, bronchial, phrenic and pericardiacophrenic arteries. In slow occlusion of coronary arteries, there may be a reversal of blood flow along the anterior cardiac veins and smallest cardiac veins (venae cordis minimae) to the myocardium from the heart chambers. **More than one artery** may be involved in myocardial infarction. Myocardial infarction is caused by atherosclerosis.

Venous drainage of the heart
The venous blood from the wall of the heart is drained mainly by the *coronary sinus*. The coronary sinus opens into the right atrium. The **coronary sinus** has many tributaries.
- Great cardiac vein
- Middle cardiac vein
- Oblique vein of the left atrium
- Left marginal vein
- Small cardiac vein

Anterior cardiac veins drain blood from the anterosuperior part of the right ventricle and drain into the **right auricle**. The smallest cardiac veins, also called **venae cordis minimae** or Thebesian veins, begin in the capillary bed of the myocardium and open in all four chambers of the heart, chiefly the atria. These are valveless veins.

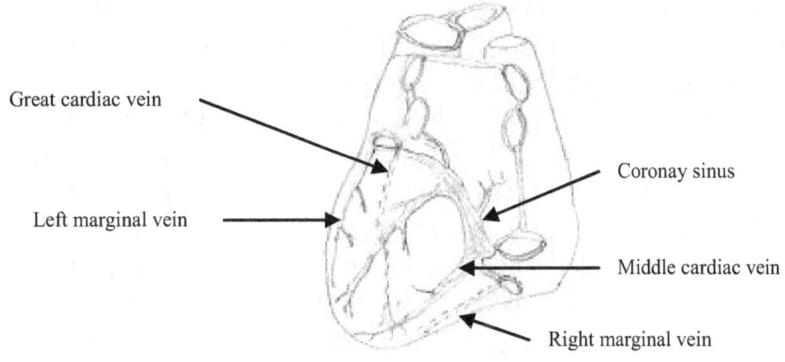

Principal veins of the heart

Innervation of the heart
Parasympathetic nerves reach the heart via the vagus nerves. These are cardioinhibitory, which means on stimulation they slow down the heart rate (**bradycardia**). Sympathetic nerves are derived from the upper five or six thoracic segments of the spinal cord. They are **cardioacceleratory**, and on stimulation they increase the heart rate (**tachycardia**) and also dilate the coronary arteries. Both parasympathetic and sympathetic nerves form the superficial and deep cardiac plexus. Visceral pain from the heart is transmitted by visceral sensory fibers that accompany sympathetic fibers and is typically referred to somatic structures such as left upper limb (referred pain). The visceral sensory fibers enter the spinal cord through the dorsal roots like the somatic sensory

fibers. Although pain from the heart is referred to the left arm, the pain may be referred to right arm, both arms, the neck and chin, or the back.

Referred pain
Referred pain is caused by visceral **nociceptive** afferent fibers that terminate on the same secondary neurons in the dorsal horn as somatic nociceptive sensory fibers. The sensory input then passes through the spinothalamic tract to the ventral posterolateral nucleus of the thalamus to the somatosensory cortex of the brain. The **brain interprets** some of the sensory inputs from the damaged heart as originating from the body not from viscera.

Cor pulmonale
Cor pulmonale is **right sided heart failure** due to lung conditions such as emphysema, chronic bronchitis, or cystic fibrosis etc. There is high blood pressure in the pulmonary circulation and in the right ventricle in cor pulmonale.

Fetal circulation
The blood from the placenta, which is **rich in oxygen**, reaches the fetus through the **umbilical veins**. The inferior vena cava receives blood from the umbilical vein, but also from the portal vein via the ductus venousus. Oxygenated blood then flows from the inferior vena cava to reach the right atrium. Blood in the right atrium either reaches the left atrium through the foramen ovum or it reaches the right ventricle through the tricuspid valve (right atrioventricular valve). Blood in the right ventricle exits through the pulmonary trunk and reaches the arch of the aorta through the **ductus arteriosus**. Blood from the left atrium (collect in the left atrium from the right atrium through the **foramen ovale**) reaches the left ventricle through the mitral valve (left atriventricular valve). Blood from the left ventricle comes out through the ascending aorta, arch of the aorta, and descending thoracic aorta, which continues as the abdominal aorta. Blood from the aorta reaches the internal iliac arteries. The **umbilical artery** receives de-oxygenated blood returning from the fetus to the placenta.

The right atrium also receives blood from the Superior Vena cava. The left atrium also receives very little blood from the pulmonary veins.

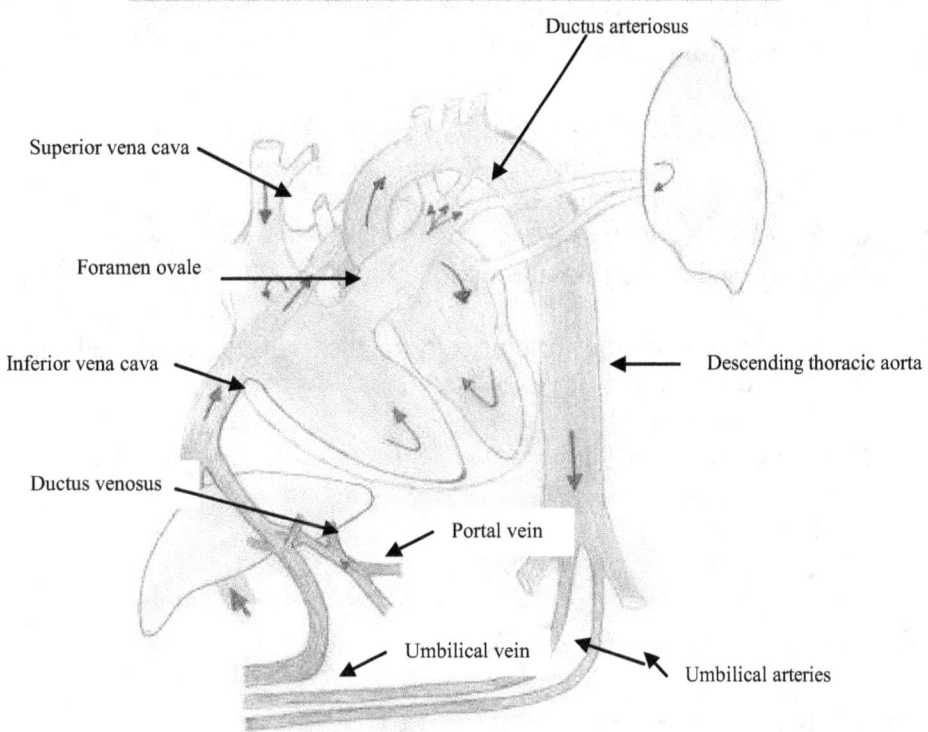

Fetal Circulation

The fetal/embryonic structures and their adult represntations

Fetal Structure	Adult Structure
Left Umbilical Vein	Ligamentum Teres Hepatis
Umbilical Arteries	Medial Umbilical Ligaments and Superior Vesical Artery
Ductus Arteriosus	Ligamentum Arteriosum
Ductus Venosus	Ligamentum Venosum
Foramen Ovale	Fossa Ovalis
Allantois, Urachus	Median Umbilical Ligament
Notochord	Nucleus Pulposus
Septum secundum	Limbus fossa ovalis

Objective Questions (Set-16)
1.   Compare the fetal structure with that of the adult.

Multiple Choice Questions (Set-16)

1.   Which of the following structures is the remnant of the right umbilical artery?
A. Right internal iliac artery
B. Right common iliac artery.
C. Right medial umbilical ligament.

    D. Ligamentum teres hepatis.

    E. Ligamentum venosum

2.   Which of the following circulatory changes take place at birth?
    A. Cessation of blood through the ductus arteriosus
    B. Flow of blood through the foramen ovale
    C. Increased right atrial pressure
    D. Decreased blood flow through the lung

3.   Which of the following structures forms the right border of the heart in the Plane X-Ray P-A View?
    A. Pulmonary trunk
    B. Arch of the aorta
    C. Right auricle
    D. Right atrium
    E. Left auricle

MCQ (Set-16) Answers: 1. C; 2. A; 3. D

Congenital heart diseases

Patent Ductus Arteriosus (PDA)
Ductus Arteriosus connects the left branch of the pulmonary trunk to the arch of the aorta in the fetus. After birth, it becomes the ligamentum arteriosum. Patent Ductus Arteriosus (PDA) after birth is diagnosed by continuous **machine like murmur**. It is a left to right shunt as characterized by cyanosis in the lower extremities (blue coloration of the skin due to increased deoxygenated hemoglobin). PDA is a common congenital anomaly associated with maternal rubella and high mountain living.

Ventricular Septum Defect (VSD)
Ventricular Septum Defect (VSD) is the **most common** of congenital heart defects. It may be an isolated anomaly or a part of the **Fallots tetralogy**.
Tetralogy of Fallot is a syndrome including pulmonary stenosis, right ventricular hypertrophy, interventricular septal defect, and dextroposition and overriding of the aorta. VSD is associated with defective formation of the endocardial cushion or the interventricular septum. VSD most commonly involves the membranous part of the interventricular septum.

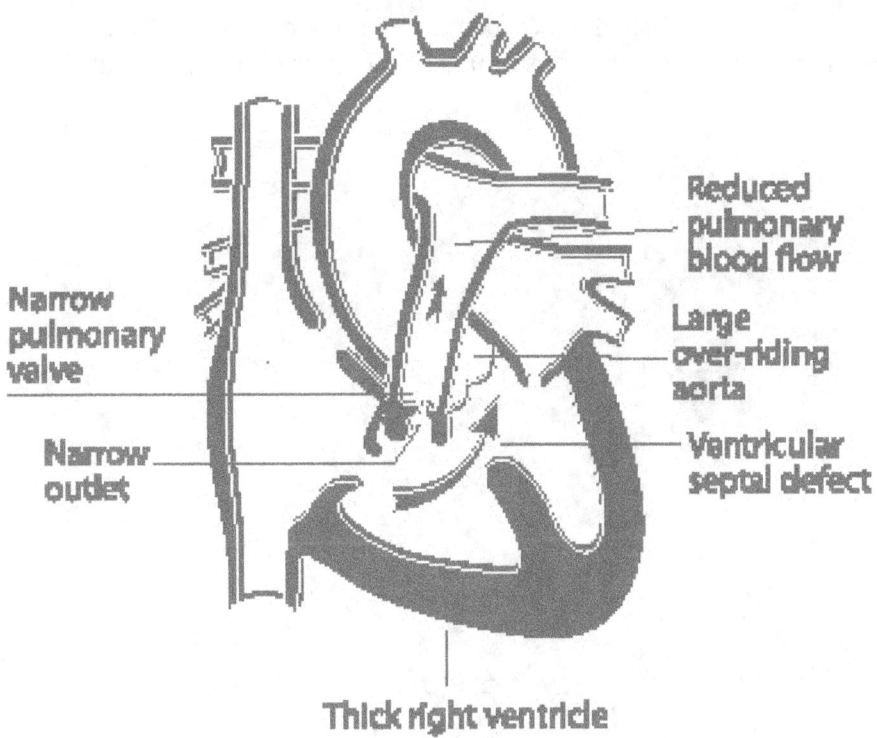

Figure: Fallot's Tetralogy 1. Pulmonary stenosis 2. Ventricular septal defect 3, Right ventricular hypertrophy 4. Dextroposition and overriding of the aorta

Atrial Septal Defect (ASD)

Atrial Septal Defect is a congenital anomaly due to incomplete closure of the **foramen ovale**. The result is a hole in the interatrial septum. A **probe-size patency** is present in 15-20% of adults but bears no clinical importance. In large ASD, the oxygenated blood from the left atrium enters the right atrium and right ventricle. The pulmonary trunk is dilated along with hypertrophy of the right atrium and right ventricle. ASD is caused by defective development of septum secundum and endocardial cushion. *During cardiac catheterization the catheter may slip from the right atrium to the left atrium through a patent foramen ovale.*

Coarctation of the aorta

Coarctation of the Aorta is a **narrowing** of the aorta distal to the origin of the left subclavian artery, close to the ductus arteriosus. There is **hypertension** in the upper extremity with high volume pulse and **hypotension** in the lower extremity with feeble pulse. There may be associated leg **cramps and nosebleed**. Mild coarctation of the aorta is compatible with life. X-Ray reveals figure **of "3"**.

Collateral circulation is established to compensate the blood flow to the legs. Surgical correction is recommended depending on the interruption of blood flow.

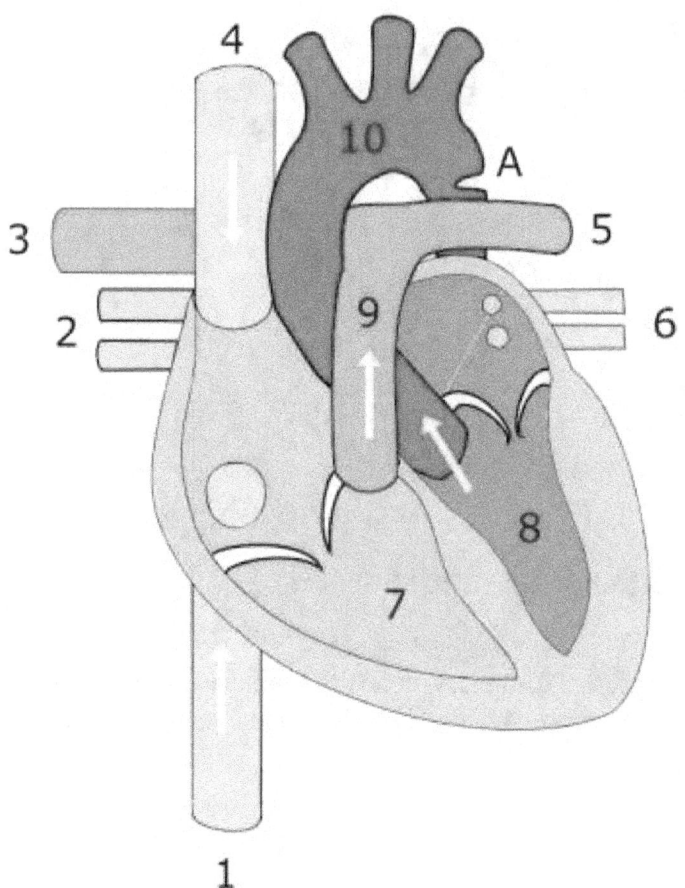

Figure: showing heart with coarctation of the aorta. **A: Coarctation (narrowing) of the aorta.** 1:Inferior vena cava, 2:Right pulmonary veins, 3: Right pulmonary artery, 4:Superior vena cava, 5:Left pulmonary artery, 6:Left pulmonary veins, 7:Right ventricle, 8:Left ventricle, 9:Pulmonary artery, 10:Aorta

Hypertrophic Cardiomyopathy

This is a familiar cause of sudden cardiac death in children, adolescents, and in athlets.About 10% of these cardiomyopathies are congenital and are transmitted as autosomal dominant disorder. There is marked left ventricular hypertrophy often with a massively thickened interventricular septum, atrial enlargement, and a small left ventricular cavity. The hypertrophic changes possibly lead to sudden death as a result of unstable myocardial function and ventricular tachyarrhythmia's.

Dilated Cardiomyopathy

Dilated cardiomyopathy is more common than the hypertrophic cardiomyopathy.The heart is enlarged, symmetrical biventricular hypertrophy, and four chamber cardiac dilatation may lead to relative thinning of the ventricular wall.

Objective Questions (Set-17)

1. What is precordium?
2. Describe the circulation of blood through hear and lung.
3. What is the anatomical location of the apex of the heart?
4. Where does a physician auscultate apex beat?
5. Where can you feel the apex beat in a person with dextrocardia?
6. What is situs inversus?
7. What are the three layers of the wall of the heart?
8. What is coronary sulcus?
9. What are the contents of the coronary sulcus?
10. What is sinus venarum?
11. What vessels open into the sinus venarum?
12. Which chamber of the heart mostly forms the sternocostal surface of the heart?
13. Which chamber of the heart mostly forms the diaphragmatic surface of the heart?
14. Which chamber of the heart mostly forms the base of the heart?
15. Left recurrent laryngeal nerve is the branch of which nerve?
16. How are the arch of the aorta and the ligamentum arteriosum related to the left recurrent laryngeal nerve?
17. What blood vessels do the left and right recurrent laryngeal nerves wind around?
18. What is the affect of iatrogenic lesion of the recurrent laryngeal nerves?
19. Where are the trabeculae carne and pectinate muscles found?
20. What is the blood supply of the interventricular septum?
21. What is the function of the papillary muscles?
22. What is cardiac skeleton? How is the cardiac skeleton formed? What are the functions of the cardiac skeleton?
23. How is an artificial pace maker implanted?
24. What is the blood supply of the heart? What are the characteristics of the coronary arteries? What is cardiac arrhythmia? What is the cause of cardiac arrhythmia?
25. What do you mean by area of superficial cardiac dullness?
26. Describe the blood supply of the heart. What is a myocardial infarction? How does slow ischemic heart disease establish collateral circulation? Is it possible to have reversal of blood flow along specific cardiac veins?
27. What are locations of the a. S-A node b. A-V node and c. Purkinje fibers? What is the blood supply of the conducting system of the heart?
28. What is referred pain? Why is the pain from a myocardial infarction referred to the left arm?
29. What structure connects the left pulmonary artery (near the bifurcation of the pulmonary trunk) to the arch of the aorta?

30. How many pulmonary arteries and pulmonary veins are present in human body?
31. What type of blood is carried by the pulmonary veins?
32. What is the parasympathetic innervation of the heart?
33. What are the components of the Tetralogy of Fallot?
34. Define cor pulmonale. What are the causes of cor pulmonale?
35. What are the boundaries and contents of the triangle of Koch?

Multiple Choice Questions (Set-17)

1. Which of the following chambers of the heart form the right pulmonary surface of the heart?
   A. Right atrium
   B. Right ventricle
   C. Left atrium
   D. Left ventricle

2. The transverse pericardial sinus is located_____
   A. behind the left atrium
   B. inside the right ventricle
   C. between the heart and the central tendon of the diaphragm
   D. between the ascending aorta and pulmonary trunk in front, and the left atrium and SVC behind

3. A 23-year-old man was killed by a stingray while swimming in the Atlantic Ocean near Daytona Beach shore. The 6- inch sting penetrated his chest wall along the left 5th intercostal space near the sternal margin. Which of the following structures had been punctured in this accident?
   A. Left atrium
   B. Right ventricle
   C. Arch of the aorta
   D. Left ventricle
   E. Ascending aorta

4. A freshman medical student tried to palpate the apex beat of his roommate. In which of the following locations can he feel the best apex beat?
   A. Left 2nd intercostal space near the sternal margin
   B. Right 3rd intercostal space near in the midclavicular line
   C. Right 7th intercostal space on the midaxillary line
   D. Left 4th or 5th intercostal space 6 to 10 cm from the midsternal line

5. Thrombi dislodged from the left atrium cannot cause _____ embolism.
   A. coronary
   B. pulmonary

C. renal

D. cerebral

6. The smooth walled part of the left atrium is formed from the
_____.
   A. primitive atrium
   B. sinus venosus
   C. absorption of the pulmonary veins
   D. both A and B

7. Which of the following valves has two cusps?
   A. Mitral valve
   B. Aortic valve
   C. Pulmonary valve
   D. Right atrioventricular valve

8. Which of the following blood vessels has no valves?
   A. Pulmonary trunk
   B. Ascending aorta
   C. Superior vena cava
   D. Coronary sinus
   E. Inferior vena cava

9. To perform the commissurotomy in mitral stenosis, a cardiac surgeon
approaches to the mitral valve through the _____.
   A. left ventricle
   B. left auricle
   C. interatrial septum
   D. left atrium between the pulmonary veins
   E. membranous part of the interventricular septum

10. Oxygenated blood is returned to the left atrium by the
_____.
   A. coronary sinus
   B. anterior cardiac veins
   C. pulmonary veins
   D. Superior vena cava

11. Which of the following hormones is secreted from the right atrial muscles?
   A. Growth hormone
   B. Prolactin
   C. ACTH
   D. ANP

12. Where is the location of the Sinoatrial node?
   A. Right atrium

B. Right ventricle
C. Left atrium
D. Left ventricle

13. Which of the following is the only bridge between the atrial and ventricular myocardium?
A. SA node
B. AV node
C. AV bundle
D. Purkinje fibers

14. Which of the following heart chamber has supraventricular crest?
A. Right atrium
B. Left atrium
C. Right ventricle
D. Left ventricle

15. Which of the following structures is the first to receive blood from the heart?
A. Brain
B. Head and Neck
C. Wall of the heart
D. Upper extremity

16. Anterior interventricular artery arises from the_____.
A. Ascending aorta
B. Pulmonary trunk
C. Right coronary artery
D. Left coronary artery

17. Which of the following arteries arises from the left aortic sinus?
A. Left coronary artery
B. Right coronary artery
C. Pulmonary trunk
D. Ascending aorta

18. Which of the following arteries runs along the inferior border of the heart?
A. Anterior interventricular artery
B. Posterior interventricular artery
C. Right marginal artery
D. Left marginal artery
E. Right coronary artery

19. Which of the following arteries usually accompanies the coronary sinus?
A. Anterior interventricular artery
B. Right coronary artery
C. Right marginal artery

D. Circumflex branch of the left coronary artery

20. Which of the following cardiac veins accompanies the anterior interventricular artery?
A. Middle cardiac vein
B. Small cardiac vein
C. Anterior cardiac veins
D. Great cardiac vein

21. Which of the following cardiac veins accompanies the posterior interventricular artery?
A. Middle cardiac vein
B. Great cardiac vein
C. Anterior cardiac vein
D. Coronary sinus
E. Small cardiac vein

22. Which of the following cardiac vein/veins may drain blood to all four chambers of the heart?
A. Anterior cardiac veins
B. Thebesian veins
C. Great cardiac vein
D. Small cardiac vein

23. Which of the following structures is found in the right atrium?
A. Papillary muscle
B. Pectinate muscle
C. Moderator band
D. Trabeculae carnae
E. Supraventricular crest

24. The interventricular septum is connected by the papillary muscle to which of the following valves of the heart?
A. Mitral valve
B. Tricuspid valve
C. Aortic valve
D. Pulmonary valve
E. Rudimentary valve of the IVC

25. Which of the following parts of the conducting system of the heart is called pacemaker?
A. S-A node
B. A-V node
C. Bundle of His
D. Purkinje fibers

26. In which of the following chambers of the heart is the electrode from an artificial pacemaker firmly fixed?
    A. Left atrium
    B. Right atrium
    C. Right ventricle
    D. Left ventricle

27. Which of the following valve stenosis causes right ventricular hypertrophy?
    A. Aortic valve
    B. Mitral valve
    C. Tricuspid valve
    D. Pulmonary valve

28. Chordae tendinae connects which of the following structures?
    A. Interventricular septum; Papillary muscle
    B. Pectinate muscle; Interatrial septum
    C. Arch of aorta; Pulmonary trunk
    D. Papillary muscle;cusp of the mitral and tricuspid valve
    E. Cusp of the semilunar valve; interatrial septum

29. Which of the following heart chambers has the thickest wall?
    A. Left ventricle
    B. Right ventricle
    C. Left atrium
    D. Right atrium

30. Which of the following histological features is seen in the cardiac muscle (myocardium)?
    A. Spindle shaped muscle fiber
    B. Intercalated disc
    C. Multiple nuclei
    D. Subsarcolemmal nucleus

31. A PCCF student was examining a 49 year old man with hypertension for last 5 years. On palpation, the apex beat of a patient was found on the left 6th intercostal space 12 cm from the midsternal line. Which chamber of the heart was likely to be enlarged in this scenario?
    A. Left atrium
    B. Left ventricle
    C. Right atrium
    D. Right ventricle
    E. Left auricle

32. During intrauterine life, blood from the left pulmonary artery reaches the arch of the aorta through which of the following?
    A. Ductus venosus
    B. Foramen ovale

C. Ductus arteriosus
D. Left umbilical artery
E. Left umbilical vein

33.   Which of the following structures is a content of the posterior interventricular groove?
A. Great cardiac vein
B. Small cardiac vein
C. Middle cardiac vein
D. LAD

34.   Trabeculae carnae is located in the _____.
A. left atrium
B. right atrium
C. pulmonary trunk
D. aorta
E. left and right ventricle

35.   Select a correct statement
A. Mitral valve has three cusps
B. Aortic valve has two cusps
C. Pulmonary valve has two cusps
D. Right atrioventricular valve has three cusps

36.   Which of the following component of the conducting system of the heart is located at the junction of the superior vena cava and the right atrium?
A. AV node
B. SA node
C. Bundle of His
D. Purkinje fibers

37. Triangle of Koch is present in the_____.
A. Left atrium
B. Rigt atrium
C. Right ventricle
D. Left ventricle

38. Which of the following part of the conducting system of the heart is located in the floor of the triangle of Koch.
A. Sinoatrial node
B. Atrioventricular node
C. Bundle of His
D. Purkinje fibers

MCQ (Set-17) Answers: 1. A; 2. D; 3. B; 4. D; 5. B; 6. C; 7. A; 8. C; 9. B; 10. C; 11. D; 12. A; 13. C; 14. C; 15. C; 16. D; 17. A; 18. C; 19. D; 20. D; 21. A; 22. B; 23. B; 24. B; 25. A; 26. C; 27. D; 28. D; 29. A; 30. B; 31. B; 32. C; 33. C; 34. E; 35. D; 36. B;37. B; 38.B

Trachea

Overview

The *trachea* or windpipe is the patent tube for passage of air to and from the lungs. The trachea is a wide tube lying in the midline, in the lower part of the **neck** and in the **superior mediastinum**. The upper end of the trachea is continuous with the lower end of the larynx. In the lower end, the trachea ends by dividing into left and right principal bronchi. The trachea is 10 to 15 cm in length. Its external diameter is about 2 cm in males and about 1.5 cm in females. The upper end of the trachea lies at the lower border of the cricoid cartilage, opposite the 6th Cervical vertebra. The **lower end** of the trachea ends at the level of the sternal angle (intervertebral disc between the T4/T5). The trachea has a fibroelastic wall supported by 16-20 C-shaped hyaline cartilage rings. Posteriorly, the gap is closed by a smooth muscle called trachealis. The esophagus is located immediately behind the trachea. The last tracheal ring has a keel like process called *carina*. It is present between the orifices of the main bronchi. The mucus membrane over the **carina** is very sensitive to bronchoscopy and is associated with cough reflex. The carina may be distorted in bronchogenic carcinoma due to involvement of the inferior tracheobronchial lymph nodes. The **lumen** is lined by pseudostratified ciliated columnar epithelium.

The **arterial supply** of the trachea is the inferior thyroid artery, a branch of thyrocervical trunk. The **venous drainage** is the inferior thyroid venous plexus. The **lymphatic drainage** is the pretracheal, paratracheal and tracheobronchial lymph nodes. The **sympathetic nerve supply** is fibers from the sympathetic trunk (vasomotor). The **parasympathetic** is through the vagus and recurrent laryngeal nerve for , secretomotor to the gland and motor to the trachealis muscle. General sensation from the mucus membrane of the trachea is carried by the recurrent laryngeal nerves.

Clinical notes on trachea

- In plane radiographs, the trachea is seen as a vertical translucent shadow due to air inside it.
- Clinically, trachea is palpated above the **suprasternal notch**.
- **Tracheostomy** is done if the airway in the larynx is obstructed by cancer or foreign body.
- The trachea may get compressed by surrounding structures and may cause **dyspnea** (difficulty in breathing) as seen in the enlargement of the **thyroid (goiter).**
- **Tracheal tug** is the downward pull of the trachea, and a downward movement of the larynx, synchronous with the action of the heart and symptomatic of aneurysm of the arch of the aorta.

Objective Questions (Set-18)
1. What types of cartilage and muscles are present in the trachea?

2. What is the lining epithelium of the trachea?
3. What is carina?
4. What is the clinical importance of the carina?

Multiple Choice Questions (Set18)

1. Which of the following statements about the extension of the trachea is correct?
   A. Atlas to T12 vertebra
   B. Axis to T12 vertebra
   C. Vertebra prominence to T5 vertebra
   D. C6 vertebra to the level of the sternal angle

2. Which of the following structures are located immediately behind the trachea?
   A. Thoracic duct
   B. Esophagus
   C. Arch of the aorta
   D. Descending thoracic aorta
   E. Brachiocephalic trunk

3. The trachea bifurcates at the level of_____.
   A. angle of Louis
   B. sternoclavicular joints
   C. xiphisternal joint
   D. 1st sternocostal joints

MCQ Answers (Set-18): 1. D; 2. B; 3. A

Esophagus

The *esophagus* is a **muscular tube** forming the food passage between the phranyx and stomach. It is about 25 cm in length. It **begins** in the neck at the lower border of the cricoid cartilage, enters the diaphragm at the level of the 10th thoracic vertebra, and **ends** by opening into the stomach at the cardiac end at the level of the 11th thoracic vertebra.

Constrictions of the esophagus

There are **four** constrictions of the esophagus along its length.

- at the beginning, 15 cm from the incisor teeth
- where it is crossed by the aortic arch, 22.5 cm from the incisor teeth
- where it is crossed by the left principal bronchus, 27 cm from the incisor teeth
- where it pierces the diaphragm, 37.5 cm from the incisor teeth

Clinical notes: 1. A swallowed entity is most likely to stop at a constricted area. 2. An ingested corrosive substance would move slowly through a constricted region hence causes more injury. 3. Constriction causes resistance during the passage of the instruments.

Arterial supply of the esophagus

The cervical part of the esophagus is supplied by the inferior thyroid artery. The thoracic part is supplied by the esophageal branches of the descending thoracic aorta. The abdominal part of the esophagus is supplied by the left gastric artery.

Venous drainage

In the cervical part of the esophagus, the venous blood drains into the brachiocephalic vein. In the thoracic part, venous blood drains into the azygos vein. In the abdominal part of the esophagus, the venous blood drains into the left gastric vein.

Nerve supply of the esophagus

Parasympathetic nerve supply of the upper half of the esophagus is the recurrent laryngeal nerve. The lower half is the esophageal plexus formed mainly by the vagus nerve. The **sympathetic nerve** supply of the upper half is the middle cervical ganglion. The lower half is T1 to T4 thoracic ganglia and splanchnic nerves. **Anterior and posterior vagal trunks** are formed from the lower part of the esophageal plexus.

Structure/Histology of the esophagus

The **lumen of the esophagus** is always closed except during the passage of food bolus. The lumen is star-shaped and is lined by nonkeratinized stratified squamous epithelium. The **submucosa** has mucus secreting esophageal glands. At the upper one third of the esophagus, the **muscular layer** consists of only skeletal muscle cells; in the middle third, a mixture of skeletal and smooth muscle cells; and at the distal end, only smooth muscle cells. The outer wall of the entire esophagus is covered by a loose connective tissue, except the abdominal part of the esophagus which is lined by the serosa.

Clinical notes on esophagus

- *Achalasia cardia* is neuromuscular incoordinatin of the lower part of the esophagus. The lower part of the esophagus does not dialate when the food bolus reaches there. There is dyphagia (difficulty in swallowing), cough, retrosternal pain, regurgitation, and vomiting of undigested food material.
- The lower part of the esophagus is one of the sites of **portosystemic anastomosis** seen in portal hypertension.
- **The esophageal varices** (formed in the submucosal layer of the esophagus due to dilatation of the venous sinuses, caused by portal hypertension) may rupture and may cause hematemesis (vomiting of blood).
- *Barret's esophagus* is epithelium of the lumen of the lower third of the esophagus changed to columnar due to exposure to gastric contents in GERD (gastro esophageal reflux disease). Barrets esophagus may warn that cancer may present.
- *Boerhaave's esophagus* is the rupture of the esophagus seen in bulimia nervosa or by an endoscopy procedure.
- *Mallory Weiss Syndrome* is a linear tear in the gastro esophageal junction due to vomiting.

Objective Questions (Set-19)

1. The esophagus begins at what vertebral level?
2. The esophagus passes through which mediastinums?
3. How is the vagal trunk formed?
4. What are the constrictions of the esophagus?
5. What are the clinical importances of the constrictions of the esophagus?
6. What is the blood supply of the upper third, middle third, and lower third of the esophagus?
7. What are esophageal varices? What is hematemesis? What is the structure of the esophagus?
8. What is the histologial identifying points of the esophagus?
9. Define achalasia cardia.
10. Define Barret's esophagus.
11. Define Boerhaave's esophagus.
12. Define Mallory Weiss Syndrome.

Multiple Choice Questions (Set-19)

1. What is the lining epithelium of the esophagus?
   A. Simple squamous
   B. Simple columnar
   C. Simple cuboidal
   D. Stratified squamous
2. The esophagus is located in the_____.
   A. root of the neck only
   B. root of the neck and superior mediastinum
   C. root of the neck, superior mediastinum, and posterior mediastinum
   D. root of the neck, superior mediastinum, posterior mediastinum, and abdomen

MCQ (Set-19) Answers: 1. D; 2. D

Thoracic duct

The ***thoracic duct*** is the largest lymphatic vessel in the body at approximately 45 cm in length. The thoracic duct **extends** from the lower border of the T12 vertebra or thoracolumbar intervertebral disk, as a continuation of the cisterna chyli in the abdomen to the junction between the left brachiocephalic vein and left internal jugular vein (left venous angle). ***Cisterna chyli*** is a dilated lymphatic channel irregularly present along the right side of the L1 and L2. The thoracic duct drains all lymph below the diaphragm, left half of the head/neck, and left thorax. It is a content of both the posterior and superior mediastinum. Thoracic duct has multiple valves hence it has beaded appearance. It enters the thorax from the abdomen through the aortic opening of the diaphragm and ascends between the azygos vein and the esophagus. It is medial to the descending thoracic aorta. Hemiazygos and accessory hemiazygos veins cross behind thoracic duct to reach the azygos vein.

Mnemonic: A duck (thoracic duct) passes between two geese (azy**gos** vein and esophagus)

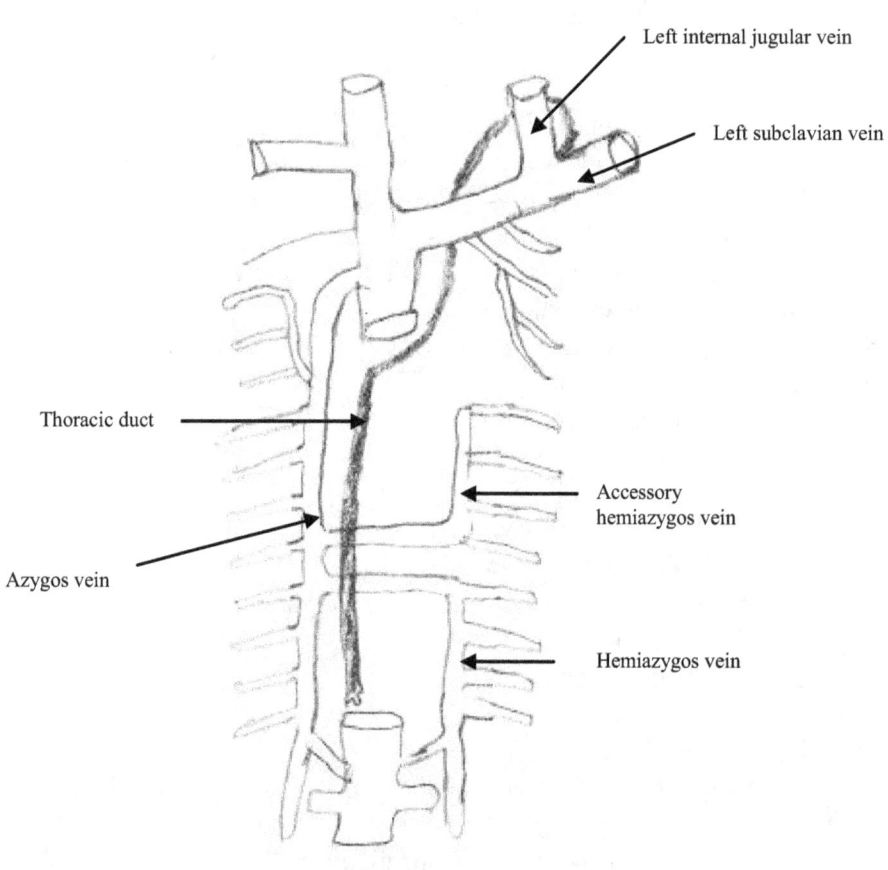

Thoracic duct

The thoracic duct is thin walled and has a beaded appearance because of its numerous valves. It is medial to the azygos vein, on the anterolateral surface of the lower thoracic vertebrae. It crosses from right to left side at the level of T4, T5, or T6. It enters the superior mediastinum and terminates at the junction between the left internal jugular vein and left subclavian vein (left venous angle). The thoracic duct receives branches from the middle and superior intercostal spaces of sides, posterior mediastinal structures, jugular, subclavian, and bronchomediastinal lymphatic trunks.

Right lymphatic duct is a lymphatic channel which drains lymph from the right half of the head, neck, and chest, and enters into the junction between the right internal jugular vein and right subclavian vein (right venous angle).

Clinical notes on thoracic duct
- Damage to the thoracic duct causes ***chylothorax***.

Objective Questions (Set-20)
1. From where does the thoracic duct begin and end?
2. What is right lymphatic duct?
3. What is cisterna chiyli and chylothorax?
4. From which areas do the thoracic duct and right lymphatic duct drain lymph?
5. The thoracic duct is located in which mediastinum?
6. Why does the thoracic duct have a beaded appearance?

Multiple Choice Questions (Set-20)
1. Select a correct statement about the thoracic duct.
   A. The thoracic duct drains lymph from the right side of the head and neck.
   B. The thoracic duct has no valve.
   C. The thoracic duct is lateral to the DTA.
   D. Hemiazygos and accessory hemiazygos veins cross behind thoracic duct to open into the azygos vein.
2. A 48-year-old man had a history esophageal resection due to cancer of the esophagus. Plane X-Ray chest on the 5th postoperative day revealed pleural effusion on the right side. Tapping of the chest revealed milky white fluid. Which of the following structures most likely damaged during the esophageal resection?
   A. Descending thoracic aorta
   B. Azygos vein
   C. Hemiazygos vein
   D. Thoracic duct
   E. Inferior vena cava

MCQ (Set-20) Answer: 1. D; 2. D

Diaphragm

The thorax is separated from the abdomen by a large, double-domed, musculotendinous partition, called the *diaphragm*, also known as the ***thoracoabdominal diaphragm***. The level of the domes of the diaphragm varies according to the phase of respiration, posture (supine or standing), and the size and degree of distension of the abdominal viscera.

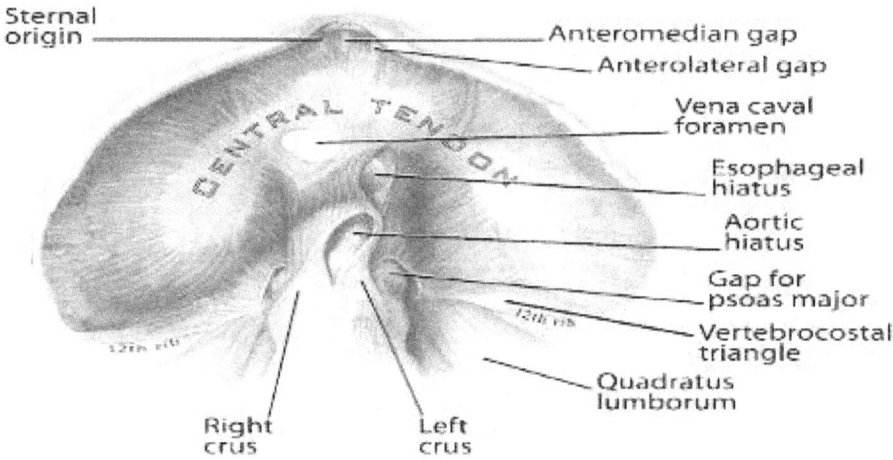

Muscular origin of the diaphragm

The diaphragm is made up of **skeletal muscle**. The muscular part of the diaphragm is situated peripherally with fibers that converge in a radial fashion on the trifoliate central aponeurotic part called the central tendon. The muscular part of the diaphragm forms a continuous sheet that is divided into three parts based on the peripheral attachments. The ***sternal part*** is two muscular slips from the posterior part of the xiphoid process. The ***costal part*** is attached to the internal surface of the inferior six costal cartilages and their adjoining ribs on each side. The ***lumbar part*** arises from lateral and medial arcuate ligaments and from the anterior surface of body of the upper lumbar vertebrae by two pillars or crura (left and right crus).

Openings in the diaphragm

There are three large and several small openings in the diaphragm that allow passage to structures from thorax to abdomen or vice versa. The **three large openings** are the aortic opening of the diagphragm, the esophageal opening of the diaphragm, and the vena caval opening to the diaphragm.

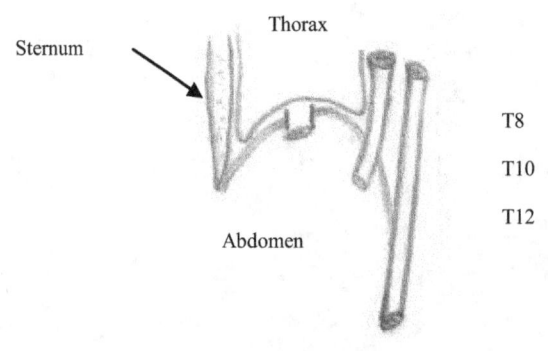

Vertebral levels of the diaphragmatic openings (apertures, hiatuses)

Aortic opening	T12 vertebra
Esophageal opening	T10 vertebra
Vena caval opening	T8 thoracic vertebra

Structures passing through the aortic aperture of the diaphragm
- aorta
- thoracic duct
- azygos vein*
- hemiazygos vein*
  *Azygos and hemiazygos veins may or may not pass through the aortic opening of the diaphragm.

Aortic aperture is an ***osseoaponeurotic*** opening hence contraction of the diaphragm does not impair the flow of blood through the aorta. The aorta passes between the crura of the diaphragm posterior to the median arcuate ligament.

Structures passing through the esophageal opening of the diaphragm
- esophagus
- anterior and posterior vagal trunk
- left gastric vessels
- lymphatic vessels
-

Esophageal opening is ***muscular***. The **fibers of the right crus** of the diaphragm form a sphincteric hiatus for the esophagus at the T10 vertebral level.

Structures passing through the vena caval aperture of the diaphragm
- inferior vena cava
- terminal branches of the righr phrenic nerve
- lymphatic vessels

Vena caval opening of the diaphragm is located at the junction of the right leaf with the central area of the central tendon. The inferior vena cava is **adherent** to the margin of the opening; therefore, when the diaphragm contracts during inspiration, **it widens the opening and dilates the inferior vena cava.**

There are two lesser apertures in each crus of the diaphragm for the greater splanchnic nerve and lesser splanchnic nerve.

The sympathetic trunk enters the abdominal cavity behind the diaphragm, deep to the medial arcuate ligament.

Blood supply of the diaphragm

	Superior Surface of Diaphragm	Inferior Surface of Diaphragm
Arterial supply	Superior phrenic arteries Branches of descending thoracic aorta Musculophrenic artery Pericardiacophrenic artery Branches of the internal thoracic artery	Inferior phrenic arteries Branches of the abdominal aorta

Venous drainage	Musculophrenic vein Pericardiacophrenic veins Tributaries of the internal thoracic vein Right superior phrenic vein opens into the inferior vena cava	Left and right inferior phrenic veins open into the inferior vena cava. Left inferior phrenic vein may also drain into the left renal or suprarenal vein

Nerve supply of the diaphragm

Motor innervation	Sensory innervation
Phrenic nerve	Intercostal nerves (T5-T11) and the subcostal nerve (T12) at the pheripheral part of the diaphragm At the central part of the diaphragm by the phrenic nerve

Lymphatic drainage of the diaphragm

The phrenic nodes to the parasternal and posterior mediastinal nodes drain the superior surface of the diaphragm. The inferior surface is drained by the superior lumbar lymph nodes.

Development of the diaphragm

The diaphragm develops from four components:
- Septum Transversum - Central Tendon of the Diaphragm
- Pleuroperitoneal membrane
- Muscular component of the body wall
- Dorsal mesentery of the esophagus - Crura of the Diaphragm

Diaphragmatic Hernias

A *congenital diaphragmatic hernia* develops due to left posterolateral defect. The incidence is once in 2200 newborns. The abdominal contents enter the thoracic cavity. The abnormal intestinal sounds may be auscultated on the thorax. In most cases, severe respiratory distress is seen, which includes cyanosis and dyspnea.

Parasternal hernia may be present when the muscular fibers of the diaphragm fail to develop forward. A small peritoneal sac containing small intestinal loop may enter the thoracic cavity between the sterna and costal portions of the diaphragm.

Hiatal hernia is a type of diaphragmatic hernias. It is due to the congenital shortness of the esophagus or congenital enlargement of the esophageal opening of the diaphragm. Hiatal hernia is the protrusion of stomach through the esophageal hiatus. Upper portion of the stomach is retained in the thorax and the stomach is constricted at the esophageal opening of the diaphragm. There are two types of hiatal hernias: the *sliding type* where a part of the fundus of the stomach and the gastro esophageal junction slides into the thorax; and *paraesophageal type* where the gastroesophageal junction is in the abdomen and a part of the fundus of the stomach is in the thorax. Hiatal hernia is associated with gastroesophageal reflux disease (GERD).

Figure: Diaphragmatic Hernias

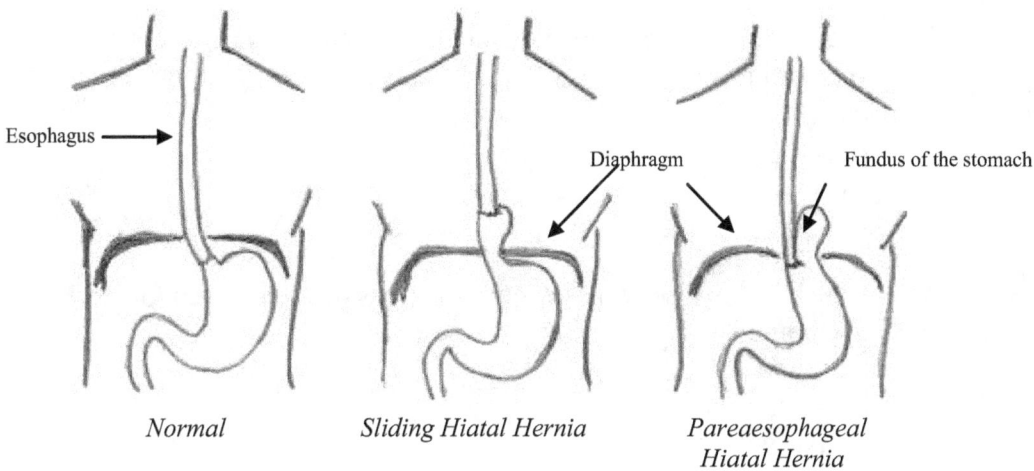

Normal *Sliding Hiatal Hernia* *Pareaesophageal Hiatal Hernia*

Mechanism and types of respiration

The diaphragm is the chief muscle of respiration. Contraction of the diaphragm and the external intercostal muscles increases the thoracic capacity and inspiration is achieved. Contraction of the diaphragm increases the vertical diameter of the thoracic cavity. The external intercostal elevate the ribs in inspiration. Normal expiration is mainly a passive process. Internal intercostal muscles work on ribs in expiration. Babies have abdominal breathing. Females have thoracic type of breathing. Males have abdominothoracic type of breathing.

Objective Questions (Set-21)

1. What is the nerve supply of the diaphragm?
2. Which bones provide muscular origin of the diaphragm?
3. What is the blood supply of the diaphragm?
4. What is the function of the diaphragm?
5. What are the hernias related to the diaphragm?
6. What is hiatal hernia?
7. What structures pass through the aortic opening of the diaphragm?
8. What structures pass through the vena caval opening of the diaphragm?
9. What structures pass through the esophageal opening of the diaphragm?

Multiple Choice Questions (Set-21)

1. Which of the following nerves innervates the diaphragm?
   A. Vagus nerve
   B. Greater splanchnic nerve
   C. Phrenic nerve

D. Thoracodorsal nerve

E. Long thoracic nerve

2. Which of the following muscles is the principal muscle of inspiration?
   A. Rectus abdominis
   B. Serratus anterior
   C. Diaphragm
   D. Latissimus dorsi

3. Esophageal hiatus of the diaphragm is located at which of the following vertebral level?
   A. T6
   B. T8
   C. T10
   D. T12

4. Which of the following structures pierces the central tendon of the diaphragm?
   A. Aorta
   B. Inferior vena cava
   C. Azygos vein
   D. Thoracic duct
   E. Esophagus

5. Which of the following structures passes behind the median arcuate ligament?
   A. Esophagus
   B. Aorta
   C. Inferior vena cava
   D. Phrenic nerve
   E. Anterior and posterior vagal trunk

6. How far does the right dome of the diaphragm reach?
   A. Upper border of the 3rd rib
   B. Upper border of the 4th rib
   C. Upper border of the 5th rib
   D. Lower border of the 6th rib

7. Which of the following structures is supported by the central tendon of the diaphragm?
   A. Left lung
   B. Right lung
   C. Superior vena cava
   D. Heart

8. Which of the following structures develops from the dorsal mesentery of the esophagus?
   A. Crura of the diaphragm
   B. Dome of the diaphragm
   C. Central tendon of the diaphragm
   D. None of the above

MCQ (Set-21) Answer: 1. C; 2. C; 3. C; 4. B; 5. B; 6. C; 7. D; 8. A

.

DIAGNOSTIC IMAGING

- CT (CAT—Computerized Axial Tomography) Scan findings
- MRI(Magnetic Resonance Imaging)
- Bone - radiopaque (white)
- Air and fat – radiolucent (black)
- Water and tissue - intermediate (grey)

In a posteroanterior view of a thoracic radiograph, the **right border** of the heart is formed by right atrium. The **left border** is formed from above downward by aortic knuckle (arch of the aorta), the pulmonary trunk, left auricle and the left ventricle.

PLEASE CONSULT www.**imagingpathways**.health.wa.gov.au/ for better conception

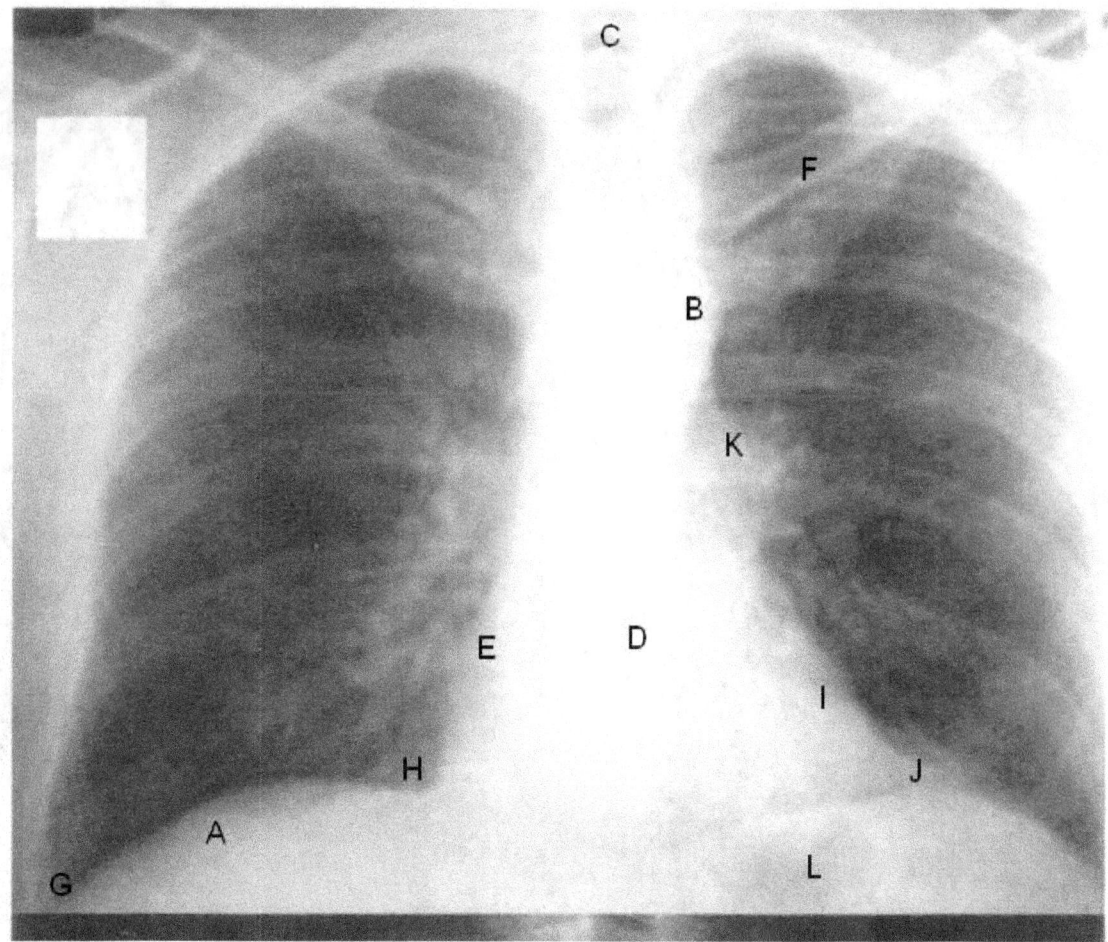

Figure: Radiograph of the Chest

A. Right dome of the diaphragm B. Arch of the aorta C. Trachea D. Right ventricle E. Right atrium F. Shaft of the left clavicle G.Right costodiaphragmatic recess of pleura H.Right cardiophrenic angle I.Left ventricle J.Apex of heart K.Pulmonary trunk and left pulmonary artery L.Fundic gas

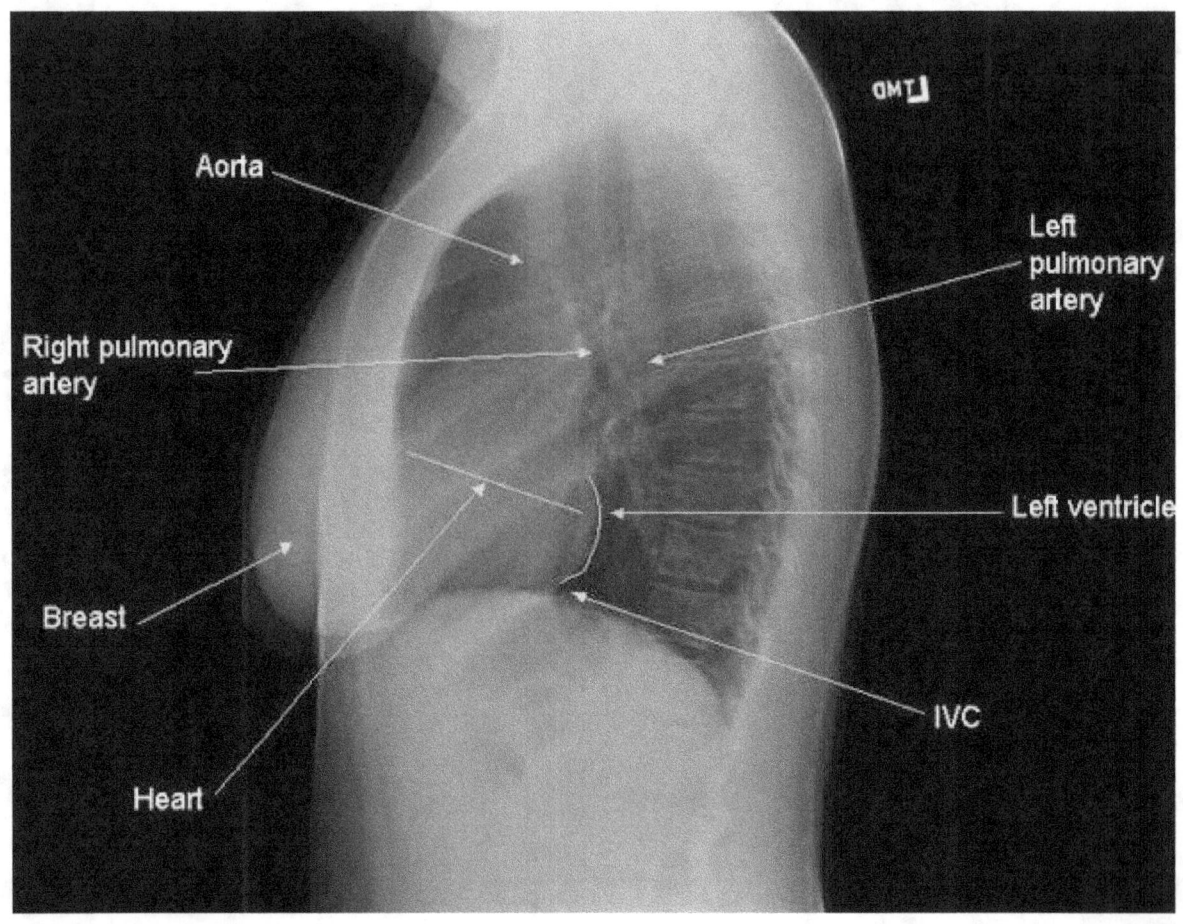

Figure: Lateral view of chest x-ray

Rule of three in the thorax (Mnemonics)

Three cavities
1. Right pleural cavity
2. Left pleural cavity
3. Pericardial cavity

Three branches of the arch of aorta
1. Brachiocephalic trunk
2. Left common carotid artery
3. Left subclavian artery

Three divisions of the parietal pleura below the thoracic inlet
1. Costal pleura
2. Mediastinal pleura
3. Diaphragmatic pleura

*Cervical pleura (cupola) extends into the root of the neck and is the fourth division of the parietal pleura.

Three lobes of the right lung
1. Superior lobe
2. Middle lobe
3. Inferior lobe
*Lobes number may vary in both the left and right lungs

Three bronchopulmonary segments in the superior lobe of the right lung
1. Apical
2. Anterior
3. Posterior

Three intercostal muscles
1. External intercostal
2. Internal intercostal
3. Intercostalis intimi

Three cusps in the semilunal valves
- Aortic and Pulmonary Values

Three cusps in the right atrioventricular valve
- Tricuspid valve

Three splanchnic nerves
1. Greater splanchnic nerve
2. Lesser splanchnic nerve
3. Least splanchnic nerve
*Least splanchnic nerve may be absent

Three unpaired veins in the posterior thoracic wall
1. Azygos vein
2. Hemiazygos vein
3. Accessory hemiazygos vein

Figure of **Three** in the X-Ray of coarctation of aorta

Spinous process of thoracic vertebra **three** is at the level of the root of the scapular spine

Three spinal nerves contribute in the formation of the phrenic nerve (C3, C4, and C5)

Three major openings of the diaphragm (esophageal, aortic and vena caval)

Three structures pass through the aortic opening of the diaphragm (Aorta, Thoracic duct, and Azygos vein)

Three structures are present in the intercostals space (intercostal vein, intercostal artery, and intercostal nerve

Check List for Gross Anatomy Lab--1
5th Quarter PCCF

1. Thoracic vertebra, body, vertebral foramen, vertebral arch, spine, pedicle, lamina, vertebral notch, articular processes, and intervertebral foramen. Atypical thoracic vertebrae-T1 (Body cervical in type, superior costal facet is complete, spine long and horizontal), T9, T10,T11, & T12—they have superior costal facets only. The transverse process of 12th thoracic vertebra has three tubercles.

2. Rami communicans in the cervical and thoracic regions

3. Curvatures of the vertebral column, Kyphosis and Scoliosis

4. Ribs---parts of a typical rib, costal groove, longest rib(7th rib), obliquity of ribs(maximum at the 9th rib), vertebrosternal ribs, vertebrochondral ribs, intercostals spaces, angle of a rib
    The 10th rib closely resembles a typical rib, but is is shorter and has only a single   facet on the head, for the body of the 10th thoracic vertebra

5. First rib, articulates with the body of the 1st thoracic vertebra, origin of subclavius, and scalene anterior muscle

6. Cervical rib

7. Bifid rib

8. Floating ribs, typical ribs(3rd to 9th ribs), true ribs, false ribs

9. Intervertebral disc

10. Articulation of the rib to the vertebra, crest of the head, intra-articular ligament, radiate ligament, costotransverse ligament

11. Sternum ,parts, xiphoid process
12. Origin of muscles from the anterior surface of the sternum—pectoralis major and sternocleidomastoid muscle. Posterior surface—Sternocostalis, sternohyoid , and sternothyroid, and diaphragm(xiphoid process).

13. Sternal angle

14. Costal cartilages

15. Jugular notch/suprasternal notch

16. Sternoclavicular joint and acromioclavicular joint

17. Coracoid process

18. Mediastinum

19. Thoracic apertures/ inferior and superior

20. The diaphragm

21. Costal margin

22. Pleural cavity

23. Costodiaphragmatic recess of pleura

24. Pneumothorax

25. Xiphisternal joint

26. Synchondrosis

Check List for Gross Anatomy Lab--2
5th Quarter PCCF

1. Identification of vertebral spinous processes—Vertebra prominence(C7), T1, T3 and the root of the spine of the scapula, T7 and the inferior agle of the scapula. The spinous process of vertebra T12 is level with the midpoint of a vertical line between the inferior angle of the scapula and the iliac crest

Attachment of ligamentum nuchae? Dermatomes over the clavicle, nipple, and xiphoid process?

2. Serratus anterior(long thoracic nerve), rectus abdominis, and external oblique(T7-T12)

3. Latissimus dorsi , deltoid muscle, coracobrachialis, biceps brachii, and subclavius

4. Stellate ganglion, ligamentum denticulatum

5. Internal thoracic artery, termination and its branches

6. Anterior and posterior intercostal arteries(superior thoracic arteries, and costocervical trunk)

7. Intercostobrachial nerve and cardiac referred pain

8. Root of the lung

9. Margin and fissures of the lung

10. Deltopectoral triangle

11. Cephalic vein

12. Lateral thoracic artery

13. Long thoracic nerve

14. Musculophrenic artery

15. Superior epigastric artery

16. The diaphragm, crura, blood supply and nerve supply

17. Fissures and borders of the lung

18. Apex and lobes of the lung

19. Apex of the heart, left ventricle, left auricle, pulmonary trunk

20. Arch of the aorta and its branches

Check List for Thoracic Anatomy Lab 3 (Identifications)

1. Right subclavian artery

2. Right common carotid artery

3. Left brachiocephalic vein

4. Right brachiocephalic vein

5. Superior vena cava

6. Azygos vein

7. Ligamentum arteriosum

8. Left recurrent laryngeal nerve

9. Left and right principal bronchi

10. Secondary bronchi

11. Carina

12. Pulmonary artery(2)

13. Pulmonary veins(4-5)

14. Tributary of pulmonary vein

15. Tertiary bronchus

16. Left margin of the cardiovascular shadow—a. Arch of aorta(aortic knob) b. pulmonary trunk c. left auricle d. left ventricle e. apex of the heart

17. Right margin of the cardiovascular shadow—right atrium

18. Right and left costodiaphragmatic recess

19. Right and left dome of the diaphragm

20. Acromioclavicular joint

21. Sternoclavicular joint

22. Normal epiphysis of humerus

23. Clavicle

24. 11th and 12th ribs

Thoracic anatomy check list 4

1. Lobes, Surfaces, apex and base of the lungs

2. Horizontal fissure and oblique fissure

3. Hilum and root of the lung

4. Right lung and related structures (medial view)—Superior vena cava, Inferior vena cava, Right brachiocephalic vein, Azygos vein, Esophagus, and Cardiac impression

5. Pulmonary ligament

6. Anterior border of the left lung-Lingula and Cardiac notch

7. Structures at the root of the lung—Pulmonary veins (superior and inferior), Pulmonary artery, Secondary bronchi, and Hilar lymph nodes

8. Anterior, Posterior, and Inferior borders of the lung

9. Costal, mediastinal and diaphragmatic surfaces of the lungs

10. Left lung and related structures (medial view) ---Arch of aorta, Left subclavian artery, Descending thoracic aorta, Esophagus, and Cardiac impression

11. Azygos vein, posterior intercostal veins, Hemiazygos vein

12. Descending thoracic aorta, posterior intercosal arteries

13. Thoracic duct

14. Thoracic sympathetic trunk and Greater Splanchnic nerve

15. Lobar and segmental bronchus of the lung

16. Left and right pulmonary arteries, pulmonary trunk, and ligamentum arteriosus

17. Left and right brachiocephalic veins, Superior vena cava, Azygos vein, and Right superior intercostals vein

18. Vagus nerve, left recurrent laryngeal nerve, right recurrent laryngeal nerve, and phrenic nerve

Thoracic Anatomy Check List 5

1. Ascending aorta and its branches

2. Brachiocephalic trunk and its branches

3. Left common carotid artery

4. Left subclavian artery

5. Ligamentum arteriosum

6. Pulmonary trunk and its bifurcation

7. Left pulmonary artery

8. Right pulmonary artery(passes underneath the arch of the aorta

9. Left brachiocephalic vein

10. Right brachiocephalic vein

11. Superior vena cava

12. Left superior pulmonary vein

13. Left inferior pulmonary vein

14. Right superior pulmonary vein

15. Right inferior pulmonary vein

16. Inferior vena cava

17. Right atrium

18. Right auricle

19. Right coronary artery

20. Right marginal artery

21. Anterior cardiac veins

22. Small cardiac vein

23. Anterior interventricular artery

24. Great cardiac vein

25. Apex of the heart

26. Left ventricle

27. Right ventricle

28. Left auricle

29. Azygos vein

30. Arch of aorta

31. Coronary sinus

32. Middle cardiac vein

33. Posterior interventricular artery

34. Circumflex branch of left coronary artery with posterior left ventricular branch

35. Left posterior ventricular vein

36. Left coronary artery

37. Conus arteriosus

38. Base of the heart

39. Left marginal artery

40. Lateral diagonal branch of LAD

Thoracic Anatomy Check List 6

1. Pericardium—fibrous pericardium and serous pericardium

2. Transverse pericardial sinus

3. Oblique pericardial sinus

4. Muscular part of interventricular septum

5. Membranous part of the interventricular septum

6. Papillary muscles

7. Mitral valve

8. Tricuspid valve—cusps—anterior, posterior and septal

9. Aortic valve

10. Pulmonary valve

11. Supraventricular crest

12. Crista terminalis

13. Pectinate muscles

14. Opening of the coronary sinus

15. Fossa ovalis

16. Limbus of fossa ovalis

17. Interatrial septum

18. Trabeculae carneae

19. Chordae tendineae

20. Cusp of the tricuspid valve

21. The myocardium of the left ventricle

22. Valve of the inferior vena cava

23. Septomarginal trabecula

24. Left coronary artery

25. Right coronary artery

BIBLIOGRAPHY

1. Antevil, Blackbourne, Moore. Anatomy recall. 2nd ed. Lippincott Williams and Wilins; 2006.

2. Chaurasia's human anatomy. 4th ed. CBS; 2004.

3. Richard S. Snell ,Clinical Anatomy , , 7th edition, 2004

4. Cunningham's Manual of Practical Anatomy, G.J Romans, Volume 2;Oxford University Press;1986

5. Dorland's Pocket Medical Dictionary. 25th ed. Saunders; 1995.

6. Grays Anatomy. 39th ed. Elsevier Churchill Livingstone; 2005.

7. Grays Anatomy for Students, 1st Edition, Richard L.Drake, Wayne Vogl and Adam W.M. Mitchhell, Elsevier Churchill Livingstone,2005

8. Junqueira, Carniero. Basic histology text & atlas. 10th ed. MCQGraw Hill; 2003.

9. Moore, KL, Persaud. The developing human: clinically oriented embryology. 7th ed. Philadelphia: Lippincott Williams and Wilkins; 2006.

10. Moore, KL, Dally, AF. Clinically oriented anatomy. 5th ed. Philadelphia: Lippincott Williams and Wilkins; 2006.

11. Langman, Sadler. Medical embryology. 8th ed. Lippincott Williams and Wilkins; 2000.

12. Grant, Sauerland. Dissector. 12th ed. Lippincott Williams and Wilkins; 1999.

13. Selim Reza, The essentials of human osteology. 6th ed. Essence Publication; 2003

14. Drake et all, Grays Atlas of Anatomy,2005

INDEX*

143